First Responder
Patient Assessment

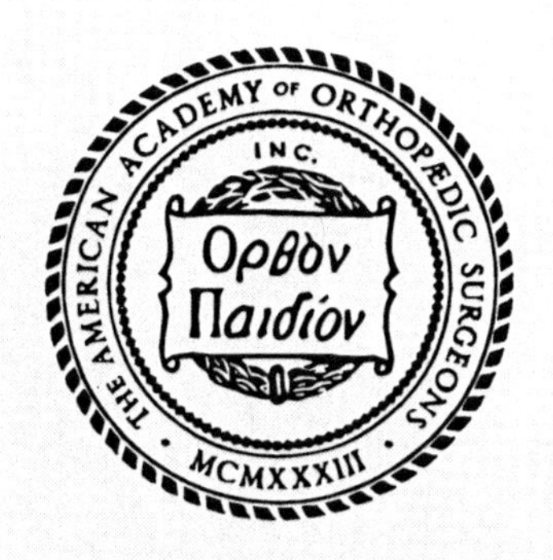

American Academy of Orthopaedic Surgeons

JONES AND BARTLETT PUBLISHERS

Sudbury, Massachusetts

BOSTON TORONTO LONDON SINGAPORE

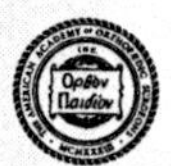

American Academy of Orthopaedic Surgeons

Editorial Credits
Vice President, Education Programs: Mark W. Wieting
Director of Publications: Marilyn L. Fox, Ph.D.
Managing Editor: Lynne Roby Shindoll
Manuscript Editor: Sharon O'Brien
Assistant Production Manager: David Stanley

Jones and Bartlett Publishers

40 Tall Pine Drive
Sudbury, MA 01776
978-443-5000
www.emtb.com
www.jbpub.com

Jones and Bartlett Publishers, Canada
2406 Nikanna Road
Mississauga, Ontario
Canada L5C 2W6

Jones and Bartlett Publishers, International
Barb House, Barb Mews
London W6 7PA
UK

Production Credits
Chief Executive Officer: Clayton Jones
Chief Operating Officer: Don W. Jones, Jr.
V.P., Senior Managing Editor: Judith H. Hauck
V.P. Sales and Marketing: Tom Manning
Senior Emergency Care Editor: Tracy Murphy Foss
Editor: Jennifer Reed
V.P. Production and Design: Anne Spencer
Senior Production Editor: Cynthia Knowles Maciel
Sales and Marketing Director: Paul Shepardson
Marketing Manager: Kimberly Brophy
V.P., Manufacturing: Therese Bräuer
Cover Photograph: Ron Olshwanger
Design and Composition: Studio Montage, Axis Print Media
Printing and Binding: Courier Company

The procedures and protocols in this book are based on the most current recommendations of responsible medical sources. The American Academy of Orthopaedic Surgeons and the publisher, however, make no guarantee as to, and assume no responsibility for the correctness, sufficiency or completeness of such information or recommendations. Other or additional safety measures may be required under particular circumstances.

This textbook is intended solely as a guide to the appropriate procedures to be employed when rendering emergency care to the sick and injured. It is not intended as a statement of the standards of care required in any particular situation, because circumstances and the patient's physical condition can vary widely from one emergency to another. Nor is it intended that this textbook shall in any way advise emergency personnel concerning legal authority to perform the activities or procedures discussed. Such local determination should be made only with the aid of legal counsel.

Notice: The patients described in "you are the cfr/emt" throughout this text are fictitious.

First Responder: Patient Assessment
ISBN: 0-7637-1651-0

Additional credits appear on page 126 which constitutes a continuation of the copyright page.

Printed in the United States of America

04 03 02 01 00 10 9 8 7 6 5 4 3 2 1

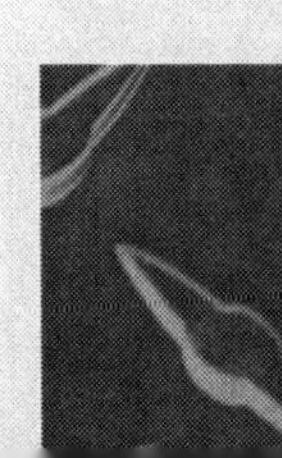

Table of Contents

Patient Assessment

Mike Smith, MICP

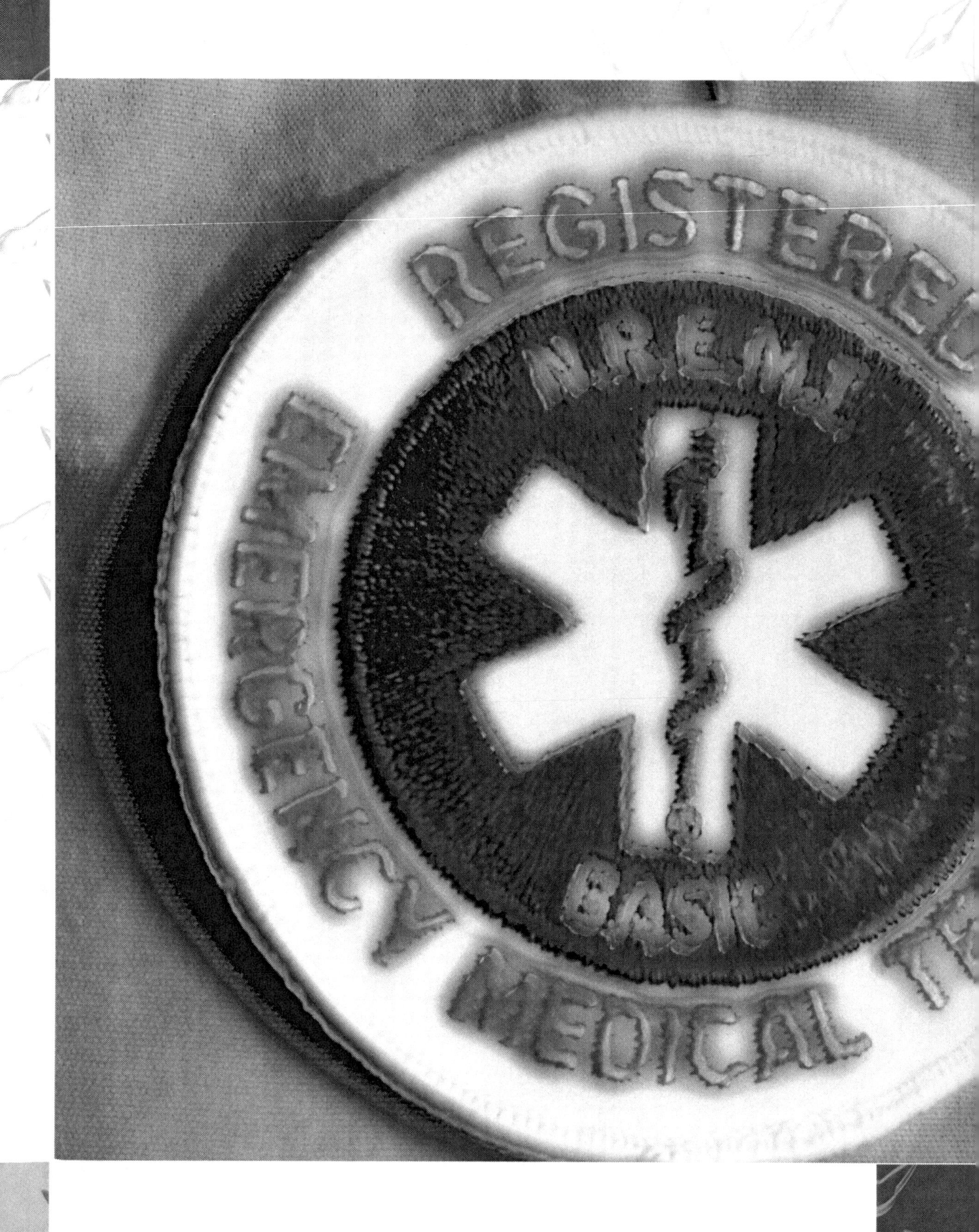

chapter 1

objectives

Scene Size-Up

Cognitive

1. Recognize hazards/potential hazards.
2. Describe common hazards found at the scene of a trauma and a medical patient.
3. Determine if the scene is safe to enter.
4. Discuss common mechanisms of injury/nature of illness.
5. Discuss the reason for identifying the total number of patients at the scene.
6. Explain the reason for identifying the need for additional help or assistance.

Affective

7. Explain the rationale for crew members to evaluate scene safety prior to entering.
8. Serve as a model for others explaining how patient situations affect your evaluation of mechanism of injury or illness.

Psychomotor

9. Observe various scenarios and identify potential hazards.

Initial Assessment

Cognitive

1. Summarize the reasons for forming a general impression of the patient.
2. Discuss methods of assessing altered mental status.
3. Differentiate between assessing the altered mental status in the adult, child, and infant patient.
4. Discuss methods of assessing the airway in the adult, child, and infant patient.
5. State reasons for management of the cervical spine once the patient has been determined to be a trauma patient.
6. Describe methods used for assessing if a patient is breathing.
7. State what care should be provided to the adult, child, and infant patient with adequate breathing.
8. State what care should be provided to the adult, child, and infant patient without adequate breathing.
9. Differentiate between a patient with adequate and inadequate breathing.
10. Distinguish between methods of assessing breathing in the adult, child, and infant patient.
11. Compare the methods of providing airway care to the adult, child, and infant patient.
12. Describe the methods used to obtain a pulse.
13. Differentiate between obtaining a pulse in an adult, child, and infant patient.
14. Discuss the need for assessing the patient for external bleeding.
15. Describe normal and abnormal findings when assessing skin color.
16. Describe normal and abnormal findings when assessing skin temperature.
17. Describe normal and abnormal findings when assessing skin condition.

(Continued)

objectives—cont'd.

18. Describe normal and abnormal findings when assessing skin capillary refill in the infant and child patient.
19. Explain the reason for prioritizing a patient for care and transport.

Affective

20. Explain the importance of forming a general impression of the patient.
21. Explain the value of performing an initial assessment.

Psychomotor

22. Demonstrate the techniques for assessing mental status.
23. Demonstrate the techniques for assessing the airway.
24. Demonstrate the techniques for assessing if the patient is breathing.
25. Demonstrate the techniques for assessing if the patient has a pulse.
26. Demonstrate the techniques for assessing the patient for external bleeding.
27. Demonstrate the techniques for assessing the patient's skin color, temperature, condition, and capillary refill (infants and children only).
28. Demonstrate the ability to prioritize patients.

Focused History and Physical Exam: Trauma Patients

Cognitive

1. Discuss the reasons for reconsideration concerning the mechanism of injury.
2. State the reasons for performing a rapid trauma assessment.
3. Recite examples and explain why patients should receive a rapid trauma assessment.
4. Describe the areas included in the rapid trauma assessment and discuss what should be evaluated.
5. Differentiate when the rapid assessment may be altered in order to provide patient care.
6. Discuss the reason for performing a focused history and physical exam.

Affective

7. Recognize and respect the feelings that patients might experience during assessment.

Psychomotor

8. Demonstrate the rapid trauma assessment that should be used to assess a patient based on mechanism of injury.

Focused History and Physical Exam: Medical Patients

Cognitive

1. Describe the unique needs for assessing an individual with a specific chief complaint with no known prior history.
2. Differentiate between the history and physical exam that are performed for responsive patients with no known prior history and responsive patients with a known prior history.

3. Describe the unique needs for assessing an individual who is unresponsive.
4. Differentiate between the assessment that is performed for a patient who is unresponsive or has an altered mental status and other medical patients requiring assessment.

Affective

5. Attend to the feelings that these patients might be experiencing.

Psychomotor

6. Demonstrate the patient care skills that should be used to assist a patient who is responsive with no known history.
7. Demonstrate the patient care skills that should be used to assist a patient who is unresponsive or has an altered mental status.

Detailed Physical Exam

Cognitive

1. Discuss the components of the detailed physical exam.
2. State the areas of the body that are evaluated during the detailed physical exam.
3. Explain what additional care should be provided while performing the detailed physical exam.
4. Distinguish between the detailed physical exam that is performed on a trauma patient and that of the medical patient.

Affective

5. Explain the rationale for the feelings that these patients might be experiencing.

Psychomotor

6. Demonstrate the skills involved in performing the detailed physical exam.

Ongoing Assessment

Cognitive

1. Discuss the reason for repeating the initial assessment as part of the ongoing assessment.
2. Describe the components of the ongoing assessment.
3. Describe trending of assessment components.

Affective

4. Explain the value of performing an ongoing assessment.
5. Recognize and respect the feelings that patients might experience during assessment.
6. Explain the value of trending assessment components to other health professionals who assume care of the patient.

Psychomotor

7. Demonstrate the skills involved in performing the ongoing assessment.

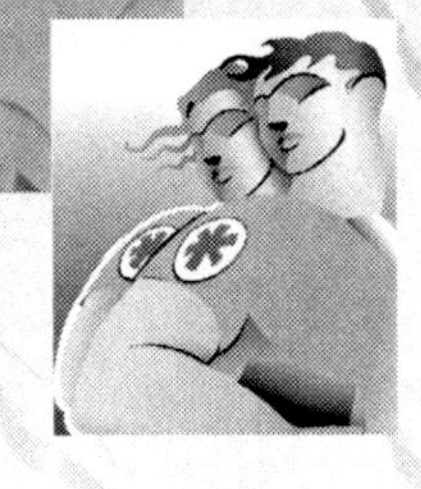

you are the cfr/emt

Squad 7 . . . Stop at the county jail lockup for "an unresponsive man." Upon arrival, you find a 24-year-old man who was thrown in the "drunk tank" last night. It's 8:00 A.M., and the patient cannot be aroused. Another man in the cell with him states that his friend had two beers and cannot be drunk. You assess the patient and find a Medic-Alert bracelet that indicates he has insulin-dependent diabetes mellitus. He most likely would have died had you not performed a thorough assessment.

Patient assessment is a skill that you will continue to refine and improve upon throughout your EMS career. This chapter will present information that you will need to build this foundation for your practice as well as help you to answer the following questions:

1. What are the goals of the initial assessment, of the focused history and physical examination, and of the ongoing examination?
2. Is an assessment needed for all patients or only for those who appear to be really sick or badly hurt?

About This Chapter

This chapter will provide a clear and comprehensive approach to Patient Assessment. A flowchart has been developed to provide a quick, visual reference to guide you through the patient assessment process. The chapter has been divided into 6 sections. Every section is color coded and numbered for easy reference. The Patient Assessment Flowchart is repeated at every section to show you "at a glance" where you are in the patient assessment process.

Special care has been taken to reflect the EMT-Basic National Standard Curriculum, but enhancement information will prepare you for your work in the field.

Scene Size-Up
Initial Assessment
Focused History and Physical Exam: Trauma Patients
Focused History and Physical Exam: Medical Patients
Detailed Physical Exam
Ongoing Assessment

Patient Assessment

From a practical point of view, prehospital emergency care is simply a series of decisions about treatment and transport. The process that guides decision making in EMS is based on your patient assessment findings. For you to make good decisions about how to best care for your patient, you must start by gathering information as you progress through the Patient Assessment process, as listed below:

- Perform the scene size-up.
- Perform the initial assessment,including stabilization of the c-spine, if indicated.
- Perform the appropriate focused history and physical exam.
- Provide rapid transport for the patient categorized as a high priority patient.
- Perform a detailed physical exam while enroute to the hospital, if indicated.
- Perform ongoing assessments.

PATIENT ASSESSMENT FLOWCHART

Scene Size-Up

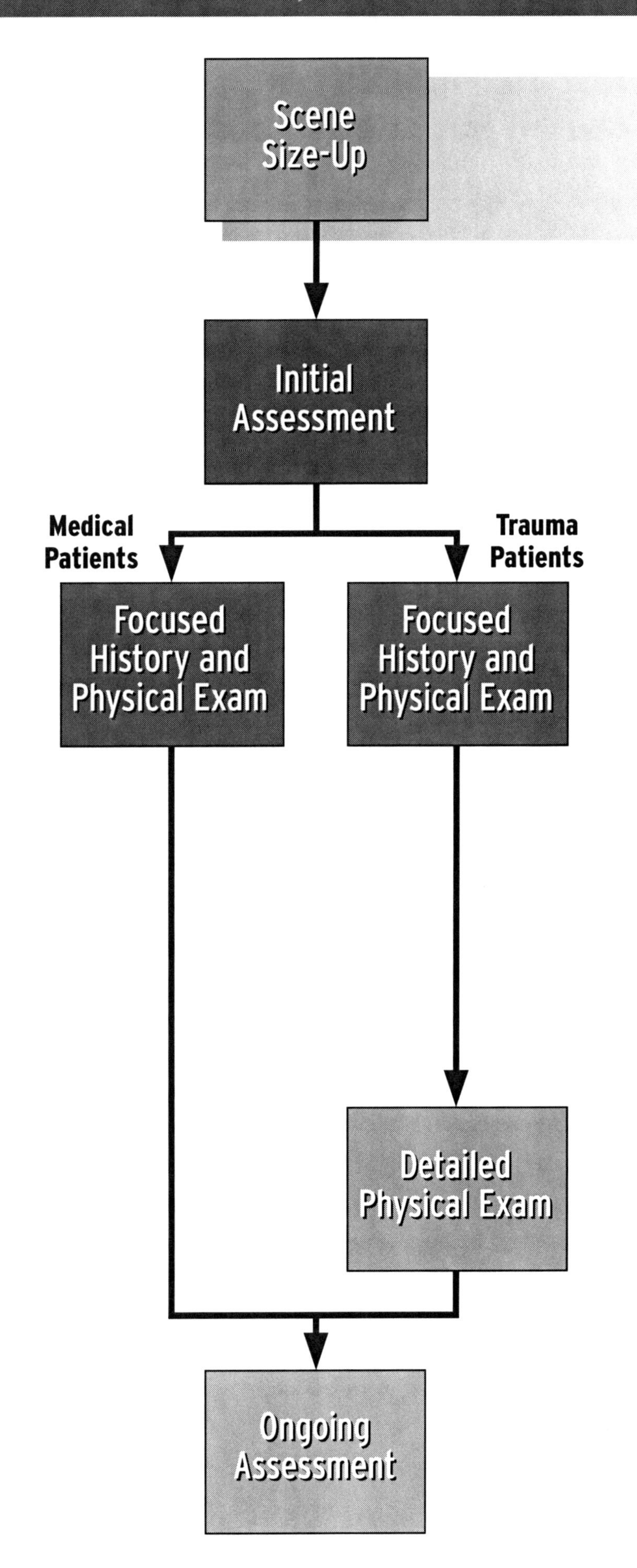

1

Dispatch Information and Mental Preparation

You should begin the assessment process long before you ever actually make contact with the patient. This *prearrival* assessment process includes using information that you learned from dispatch, as well as preparing yourself mentally to handle the call. Therefore, your first step on any call is to evaluate whatever dispatch information is available, including the location, the nature of the call, and the age and gender of the patient. While not always accurate, dispatch information may provide some insight into the following questions:

1. **What is the nature of the call and has EMS responded to the location before?** For instance, the call may be to a blind curve where head-on collisions are common. Or it may be to a long-term care facility, leading you to expect medical or traumatic problems that are common to geriatric patients.

2. **What are the likely problems based on the patient's age or gender?** These factors may help you to mentally plan ahead. For example, if you are responding to a child with chest pain, you might anticipate a traumatic injury, since this is a likely cause of chest pain in children; the same chest pain call in a 60-year-old man will likely be related to cardiac problems.

3. **What equipment or additional personnel are needed?** Often, dispatch information will help you to select the type of equipment to take to the scene. For instance, taking a backboard would be a good choice for a fall, whereas a suctioning unit, a defibrillator and a bag-valve-mask device may be useful for a patient in cardiac arrest. Dispatch to a three-car motor vehicle accident could prompt a call for additional EMS or rescue resources.

4. **What are the potential hazards?** Dispatch information can provide valuable information regarding potential hazards that you may encounter on the scene. For instance, calls related to traffic collisions may present a risk because of rapidly moving traffic on a busy highway. Calls involving fires or toxic spills can present a very real danger to rescuers through exposure to smoke or toxic chemicals. Consider these risks as you travel to the scene, and prepare a mental list of potential needs accordingly. When appropriate, consider calling for additional resources to assist at the scene.

What Is the Nature of the Call?

Suppose you are called to a long-term care facility for a woman who has fallen. The long-term care facility staff report that a 93-year-old woman fell against a door handle in the hall on her way back from lunch. They can see a large laceration on the back of the woman's head. Given this dispatch information, you should ask yourself the following questions:

- What questions would you ask the patient first?
- What type of assessment should be performed?
- What decisions need to be made in this situation?

What should you do in this situation? What should you expect? You will be confronted with the simple question of "what to do" on every call, every day.

What Are the Likely Problems?

Although it is impossible to predict what you will find with any certainty in any situation, several factors should be considered. As you learn more about different medical and trauma conditions, you will be better able to anticipate potential problems. In the above case, the patient is elderly. With that in mind, how should you prepare mentally? Next, consider possible events that might cause an elderly woman to fall, including a simple slip and fall, fainting (syncope), a cerebrovascular accident (CVA), a cardiac related event, or inadequate oxygen to the brain caused by a respiratory problem.

Once you have considered the possible causes, think about the consequences of a fall. The patient could have fractured her leg, hip, pelvis, or even spine. She could have also hit her head and/or sustained a closed head injury or a soft-tissue injury such as a laceration. Given this information, you might mentally review the signs, symptoms, and treatment of CVA, cardiac related event, or shortness of breath, as well as fractures and soft-tissue injury.

What Equipment Is Needed?

Given the information supplied by dispatch, you might take the following equipment into the long-term care facility with you:

- A blood pressure cuff and stethoscope to obtain the blood pressure, a penlight to assess the pupils, a watch with a second hand to calculate respirations and pulse.
- A long backboard, c-collar, strapping devices, and head immobilization device, in case spinal immobilization is required.
- Oxygen and all oxygen delivery equipment, including a BVM device and airway adjuncts, in case oxygen is necessary or the patient is in cardiac arrest
- Bandaging supplies, gloves, and masks whenever there is indication that a patient has open wounds

What Are the Hazards?

Finally, consider potential hazards. For the most part, long-term care facilities are usually fairly safe locations to work. Traffic should not be a problem, and—unless it is part of the nature of the call—hazardous materials should not be a problem. However, the potential for exposure to blood may present a hazard, as could angry, uncooperative family members. You should wear gloves, gowns, or masks as necessary and dictated by protocol to protect yourself against exposure to blood or other body substances.

Mental preparation is an essential part of the patient assessment process because it helps you to focus so that you are ready for any situation or circumstances at the scene. In many cases, chaos and inappropriate equipment on a scene can be traced to poor mental preparation. So use the time traveling to the scene to consider and prepare for what you are likely to find when you arrive.

Scene Size-Up

Upon arriving at the scene, it is essential to perform a scene size-up. The scene size-up is a quick assessment of the scene and the surroundings that will provide you and your partner with as much information as possible about the safety of the scene, any mechanism of injury, and/or the nature of the illness before you enter and begin patient care. Table 8-1 lists the components of the scene size-up. Your first step at any scene is to make sure that you and your partner are safe. Never become a victim yourself.

TABLE 8-1 Components of the Scene Size-Up

Safety of the Scene

- Make sure you and your partner are safe:
  - Reduce your risk of exposure to communicable disease by following BSI techniques.
  - Watch for possible dangers outside the ambulance, such as traffic, leaking fuel, downed electrical lines, fire, hazardous materials.
  - Consider your ambulance to be a relatively safe haven if you are responding to a crime scene.
- Make sure the patient and bystanders are safe:
  - Move bystanders to a safe area.
  - Ask bystanders to help with or perform a specific task.
  - Ask for additional rescuers if necessary.

Nature of the Illness/Chief Complaint

- Ask the patient, family members, or law enforcement why EMS was called.

Mechanism of Injury

- Use the mechanism of injury (MOI) as a guide to predict the type of injury sustained and to predict the potential seriousness of the injury:
  - How much force was applied to the body?
  - How long was the force applied?
  - What area of the body was involved?

Multiple Patients

- Call for additional EMS units.
- Begin triage.

Call for additional resources such as law enforcement, the fire department, rescue units, HazMat teams, and utility companies, as needed.

Body Substance Isolation

On every emergency call, you need to be sure to wear the proper personal protective equipment since this equipment will reduce your risk of exposure to communicable disease. The best way to reduce your risk of exposure is to follow body substance isolation (BSI) techniques. The concept of BSI assumes that all body fluids present a possible risk for infection.

Before you step out of the unit, you and your partner must be wearing the proper protective equipment. Vinyl or latex gloves are always indicated. Eye protection, masks, and gowns may also be indicated if there is a lot of blood or other body fluids in the patient area (Figure 8-1). Eye protection is needed when there may be a risk that blood or other body fluids will splatter or become airborne. You should put on a mask and gown, if needed and dictated by your protocol, before you enter the area immediately around the patient. If the scene involves hazardous materials or fire, wear the appropriate gear for the situation or do not enter the scene.

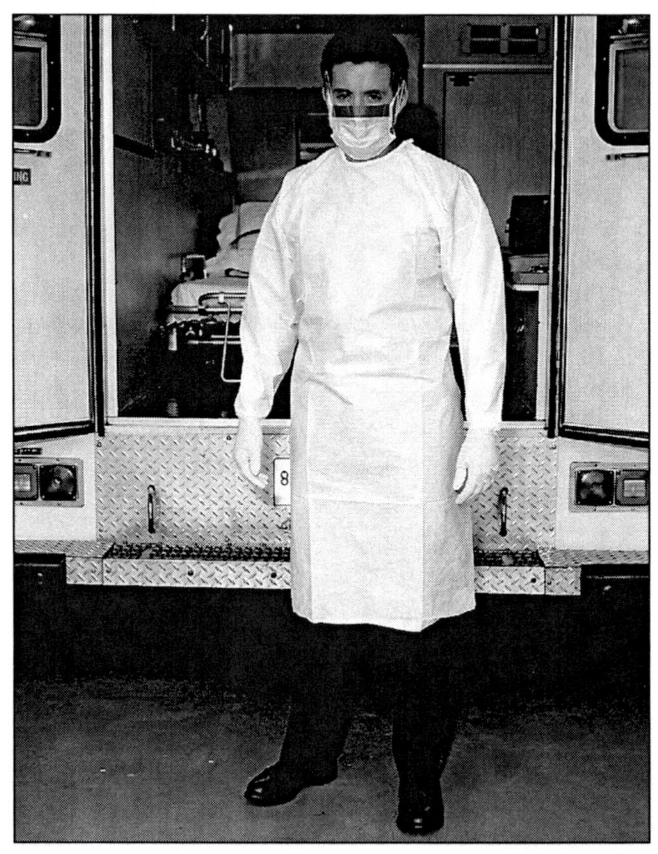

FIGURE 8-1 Proper protective equipment is vital when you are called to a scene in which there is a lot of blood or other body fluids.

Scene Safety

Scene safety is an assessment focused on ensuring the well-being of the prehospital care provider. You cannot help your patient if you become a victim yourself.

Personal Protection

Look for the following possible dangers before you step out of the unit (Figure 8-2):

- Oncoming traffic
- Unstable surfaces (e.g., wet or icy patches, loose gravel, slopes)
- Leaking gasoline or diesel fuel
- Downed electrical lines
- Hostile bystanders/potential for violence
- Fire or smoke
- Possible hazardous or toxic materials
- Other dangers at crash or rescue scenes
- Crime scenes

You should park your unit in a place that will offer you and your partner the greatest safety but also rapid access to the patient and your equipment; also be aware of egress (Figure 8-3). In many instances, law enforcement will be at the scene before you arrive. If that is the case, you should talk with them before entering the scene. Make sure to follow local protocol if the scene is a crime scene. Also be sure to have law enforcement accompany you if the patient is a suspect in the crime. Consider your unit a safe haven. You are no help to the patient if you enter the scene without first protecting yourself and your partner.

Your next concern is the safety of the patient(s) and bystanders. This is not an easy task. Bystanders can become a problem when they try to help or direct your care. Protect yourself and bystanders alike by moving them to a safe area or assigning them a specific task.

Making an Unsafe Scene Safe

Occasionally, you and your partner will not be able to safely enter a scene. This may be due to possible hazardous conditions. These situations seem very difficult when you want to provide medical care to sick or injured patients. However, your safety and that of your partner are more important. If you need more help, do not hesitate to ask for it. Be as specific as possible about the type of help you need. Remember, though, it takes time for additional resources, such as a team for disentanglement, law enforcement, or another EMS unit, to arrive at the scene.

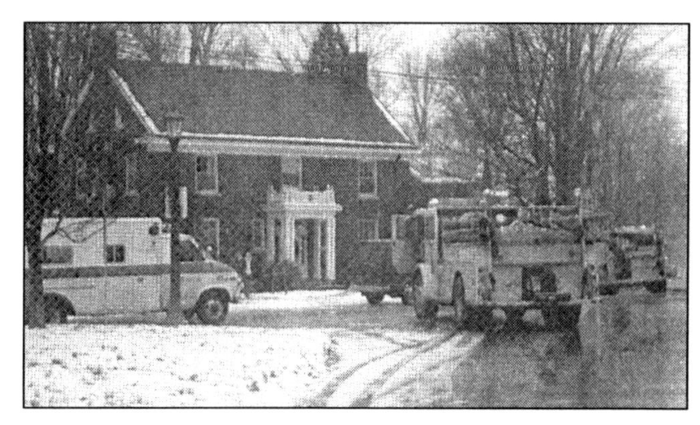

FIGURE 8-2 Before you step out of your unit, be sure to evaluate the scene for any hazards.

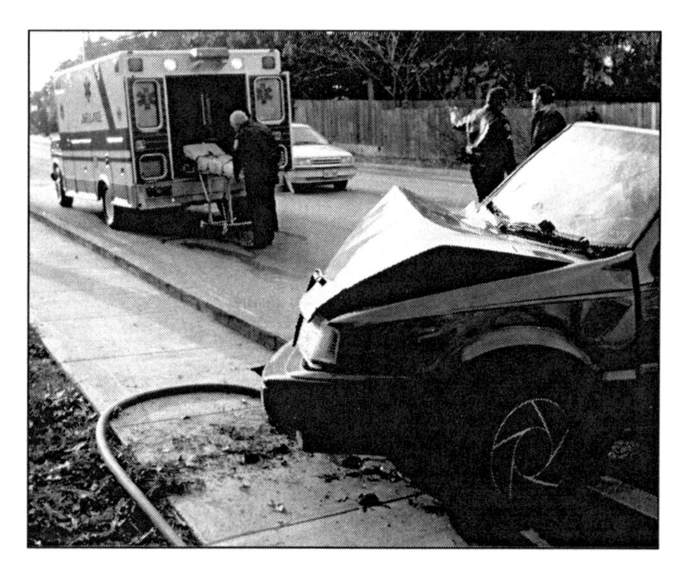

FIGURE 8-3 Park your unit in a place that is safe, yet allows for rapid access to the patient and your equipment as well as simple and swift egress. If law enforcement is already on the scene, make sure to check in with them first.

Goals of Scene Size-Up

As an EMT-B, you must ask some standard questions in all cases, whether the problem appears to be traumatic or medical in origin. Then, depending on the answers to these questions, you will ask other questions and follow other leads. But how do you begin? Prehospital assessment has four primary goals. You achieve these four goals by asking questions, obtaining answers, and responding to the information obtained. Table 8-2 lists the four goals, and the standard questions that will help you to achieve them, in order of importance and urgency.

TABLE 8-2 The Four Goals of Prehospital Assessment

The Four Goals	How to Achieve Them
1. **To identify immediately life-threatening conditions.** These conditions, such as airway obstruction, inadequate breathing, poor circulation, or grossly abnormal brain function, may kill your patient quickly. Once you identify any of these problems, you must provide interventions immediately before you perform any additional assessments.	1. **Does the patient have an immediately or potentially life-threatening condition?** If the answer is "yes," you need to start treatment by addressing the life-threatening condition and then provide immediate transport. The goal is a time-on-scene of less than 10 minutes. It should be noted that 10 minutes is considered the *ideal* amount of time spent on the scene with high priority patients. Circumstances beyond the control of the prehospital care providers can cause longer on-scene time (i.e.: serious motor vehicle accidents, building collapse, a patient pinned between a subway train and the platform, the shooting at Columbine H.S., etc.). The time spent to "correct" disentanglement or unsafe scenes does not usually include the time it takes to assess and treat the victim(s).
2. **To identify potentially life-threatening conditions.** Potentially life-threatening conditions may seriously impair or kill a patient, although they have not become serious yet. Examples include swelling in the neck that may cause airway obstruction, a respiratory condition that may worsen, or significant bleeding that—if left uncontrolled—may result in inadequate circulation (hypoperfusion). Any potentially life-threatening conditions should be closely monitored throughout the call.	2. **Is this patient sick or injured enough to require treatment?** In most cases, the answer is yes—that is why you were called. Your next step is to perform further assessment to determine what type of treatment is necessary. However, in some cases, you are called to situations that do not require emergency care. When this happens, you may simply need to provide transport. In other cases, depending upon your local protocols, you may actually leave the patient at the scene.
3. **To identify and monitor abnormalities in the patient's current condition.** Abnormalities are deviations from normal that do not present any immediate life-threats—for example, a fast pulse but a very low blood pressure. You might not identify these abnormalities initially, since your focus is on the life-threatening conditions.	3. **Does the patient require transport?** If the answer is yes, you will need to ask and answer additional questions to determine the most appropriate destination for the patient. You will also need to decide how urgently you should initiate transport.
4. **To provide information from the prehospital assessment to compare with later results.** This information is the first that you gather about the patient's condition. Your initial assessment of the patient is important because, in most cases, you are the first to evaluate a patient. All other assessments of the patient, whether they are done in the field, the emergency department, or the hospital, will be compared with this initial assessment. Changes or trends in the patient's condition may be significant in identifying developing problems. As a result, the information from the prehospital assessment often serves as a basis for making changes in treatment throughout the patient's hospital stay.	4. **How did the patient respond to treatment?** To answer this question, you must continue with your ongoing assessments. Once some form of care has been initiated, it is essential for you to reassess the patient. If the patient improves with treatment, you might wish to continue treatment as started. However, if the patient's condition becomes worse, you need to determine, through additional assessment, whether you need to change your approach to treatment.

Mechanism of Injury/ Nature of Illness

One of the great dangers in performing the prehospital assessment is giving in to the temptation to categorize your patient immediately *as either a trauma patient or a medical patient.* Remember, the fundamentals of good patient assessment do not change, despite the unique aspects of trauma and medical care. Careful evaluation of the scene, including the possible mechanism of injury and/or the nature of illness, along with the other information that you gather will help you to lean in one direction or the other. Family members, bystanders, and law enforcement can often tell you what prompted the call to 9-1-1. After you have completed your assessment, you will come to a conclusion as to whether your patient's main problem is medical or traumatic.

Determine from the patient why EMS was activated. You might also rely on information provided by family or bystanders.

Determine how many patients are involved. If there are more patients than your unit can effectively handle, initiate a mass-casualty plan. Call for additional help before making contact with patients or beginning triage. You are less likely to call for help once you are involved in patient care.

Mechanism of Injury

As an EMT-B, you will be called to motor vehicle crashes or other situations in which patients may have sustained life-threatening traumatic injuries. To care for these patients properly, you must understand how traumatic injuries occur, or the mechanism of injury. With a traumatic injury, the body has been exposed to some force or energy that has resulted in a temporary injury, permanent damage, or even death (Figure 8-4).

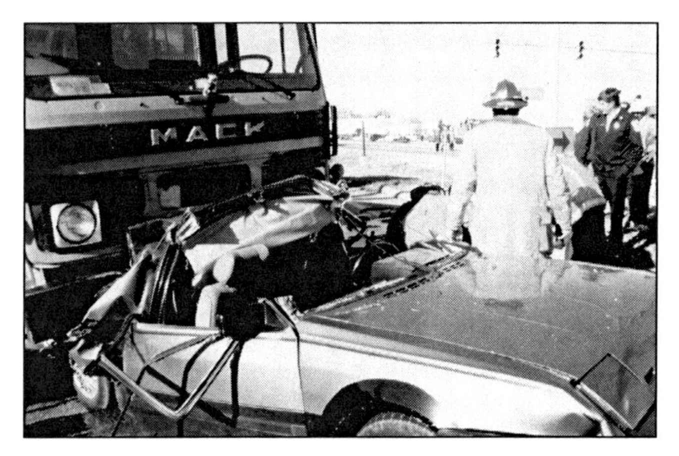

FIGURE 8-4 With traumatic injuries, the patient has been exposed to some force or energy that results in injury or even possibly death. You can learn a great deal about that force by simply looking at the mechanism of injury.

As you might expect, some parts of the body are more easily injured than others. The brain and the spinal cord are very fragile and easy to injure. Fortunately, they are protected anatomically by the skull, the vertebrae, and several layers of soft tissues. The eyes are also easily injured. Even small forces on the eye may result in serious injury. The bones and certain organs are hardier and can absorb small forces without resulting injury. The net result of this information is that you can use the mechanism of injury as a kind of guide to predict the potential for a serious injury by evaluating three factors: the amount of force applied to the body, the length of time the force was applied, and the areas of the body that is involved.

You will commonly hear the terms "blunt trauma" and "penetrating trauma" (Figure 8-5). With blunt trauma, the force of the injury occurs over a broad area, and the

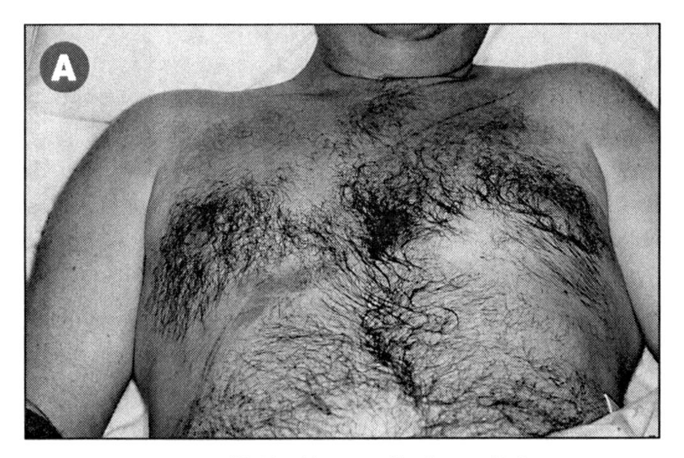

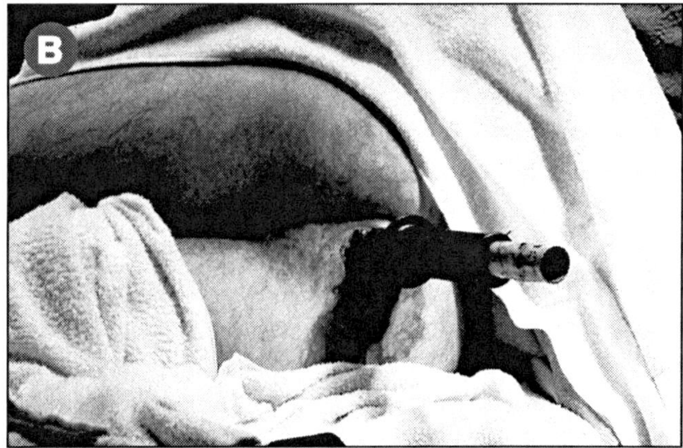

FIGURE 8-5 A: With blunt trauma, the force of injury occurs over a broad area, and the skin is not broken.
B: With penetrating trauma, an object pierces the skin and creates an open wound.

skin is usually not broken. However, the tissues and organs below the area of impact may be damaged. With penetrating trauma, the force of the injury occurs at a small point of contact between the skin and the object. The object pierces the skin and creates an open wound. The degree of injury depends on the characteristics of the penetrating object, the amount of force or energy, the part of the body affected, and the likelihood of infection.

Motor vehicle crashes. In motor vehicle crashes, the amount of force that is applied to the body is directly related to the speed of the crash. As the speed of a crash increases, the forces that are exerted on the patients increase as well. Therefore, the victim of a motor vehicle collision should be evaluated according to the area of the body that was most likely injured. Your evaluation should also be based, to some extent, on the patient's position in the car, the use of seat belts, and how the patient's body shifted during the crash (Figure 8-6). Drivers are typically at higher risk for serious injury than passengers because of the potential for striking the steering wheel with the chest, abdomen, or head. Front seat passengers may also be injured by striking the dashboard.

Risk for serious injury also varies depending on whether seat belts are used and whether they are worn properly. Unbelted victims are at much higher risk for a number of other injuries because they may be catapulted throughout the car. As they go "up and over" or "down and under," they may strike the sides, ceiling, floor, dashboard, steering wheel, or windshield. Even worse, the unrestrained victim may be ejected from the vehicle, dramatically increasing the risk of head injury, spinal cord injury, and possibly death.

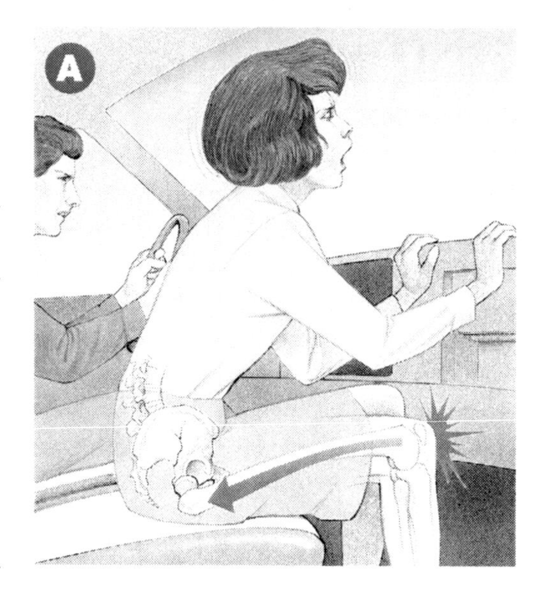

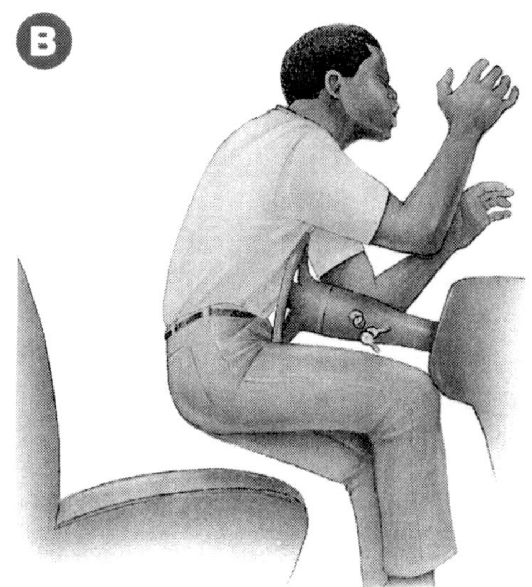

FIGURE 8-6 A: Injury to the lower extremities and pelvis can occur when the knee strikes the dashboard. **B:** Injury to the chest and abdomen occurs when the patient's chest and/or abdomen strikes the steering wheel.

Falls. In falls, the amount of force that is applied to the body is directly related to the distance fallen. However, the area of the body injured is very hard to predict. Long falls are high-force falls, and patients should be evaluated accordingly. Any patient who has fallen more than three times his or her own height, or greater than 20', should be considered at risk for serious injury. With children, a fall of 10' or more is potentially lethal.

If the patient is alert, you should attempt to determine exactly what happened during the fall. When possible, you should also identify what the patient landed on and how he or she landed. This information, which may be gleaned from the patient and/or bystanders, will help you to predict what areas of the body might be involved.

Gunshot and stab wounds. Penetrating trauma, often the result of a gunshot or stab injury, is also very difficult to evaluate because there is little external evidence of the actual damage. The amount of force that is applied to the body in a gunshot wound is most directly related to the caliber of the weapon and the distance the weapon was from the patient when it was fired. Point-blank or high-caliber gunshot wounds are high-force injuries. By comparison, the force that is exerted on the patient in stab injuries is minimal, even though these injuries can still be lethal.

The area of the body that is involved in penetrating trauma may be very difficult to predict. In gunshot wounds, the area that is involved may be predicted by

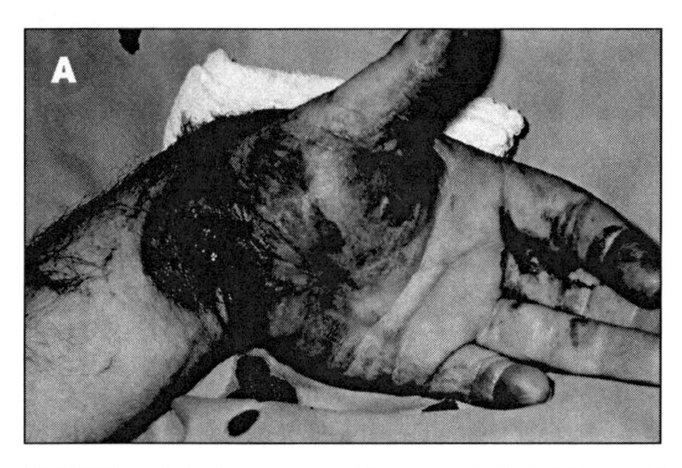

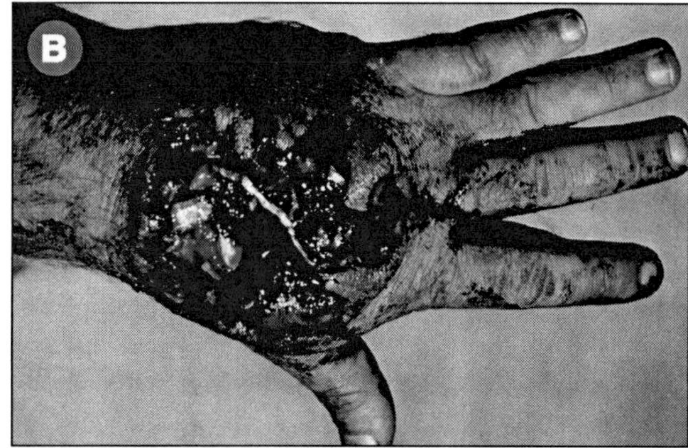

FIGURE 8-7 **A:** Entrance wound from a gunshot. **B:** Exit wound from a gunshot.

creating an imaginary line between the entrance wound and the exit wound, if one exists, although this is only an approximation at best (Figure 8-7). However, it is important to remember that bullets may bounce off dense bones or organs in the body, making the exact path almost impossible to determine. Some bullets are even designed to tumble or break apart after they enter the body.

In stab wounds, the body area that is involved can be estimated by looking at the location of entrance and the length of the instrument that was used in the stabbing, if known. Remember that you can only estimate the extent of the injury. An assailant may have moved the weapon in a back-and-forth motion after it entered the patient.

Number of patients. As part of your scene size-up, it is essential that you accurately determine the total number of patients. This determination is critical for your estimate of the need for additional resources, such as the HazMat team or a specialized rescue group. You should ask yourself the following questions when considering the need for additional resources:

- How many patients are there?
- What is the nature of their condition?
- Who contacted EMS?
- Is this a possible crime scene in which evidence may need to be preserved?
- Are hazardous materials, such as chemicals or leaking fuel, involved?
- Does the scene pose a threat to your or your patient's safety?

When there are multiple patients, you should call for additional units immediately and then begin triage (Figure 8-8). Triage is a process of identifying the severity of each patient's condition. Once that is accomplished, you can begin to establish treatment and transport priorities. One EMT-B, usually the most experienced, should be assigned to perform triage. This process will help you to provide care and allocate your personnel and equipment resources most effectively and efficiently in a multiple-patient situation. If there is a large number of patients or if patient needs are greater than the available resources, put your local mass-casualty plan into action.

In these situations, you should always call for additional resources, such as law enforcement, the fire department, rescue units, ALS, and even utilities as soon as possible. It is never wrong to call for backup, even if the extra units are sent back. Remember, you are less likely to ask for help after you begin patient care because at that point, you are part of the scene, particularly at a motor vehicle crash in which patients require spinal immobilization.

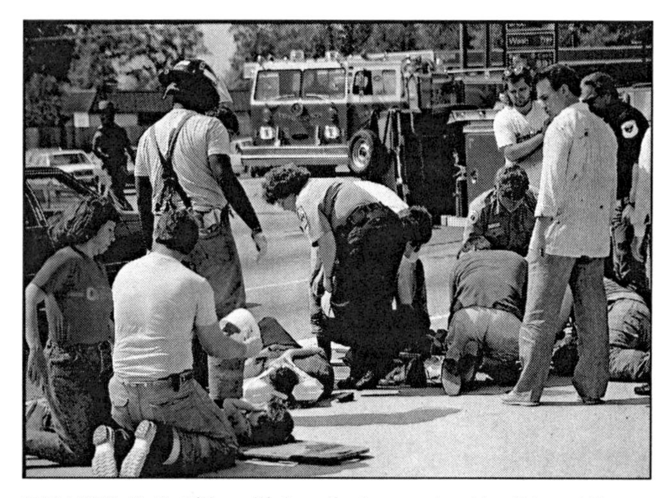

FIGURE 8-8 With multiple patients, you should call for additional resources and then begin triage.

Initial Assessment

During the prearrival and scene size-up phases, you speculated about the patient's condition, based on dispatch information, and asked and answered questions about scene safety. These steps are critically important, particularly in light of their role in ensuring your safety. However, patient assessment actually begins when you come into contact with the patient.

The patient assessment process consists of four steps:

1. The **initial assessment** helps you to identify any immediately or potentially life-threatening conditions and then begin appropriate treatment.
2. The **focused history and physical exam** help you to further evaluate the patient's major complaints or any problems that are immediately evident.
3. During the **detailed physical exam,** you gather information in situations in which the problem does not need to be readily identified or you need more specific information about problems that were found during the focused history and physical exam.
4. The **ongoing assessment** helps you to monitor problems that have already been identified and to assess the patient's response to treatment.

The initial assessment has a single, critical, all-important goal: to identify and initiate treatment of immediately or potentially life-threatening conditions. Information concerning life-threatening conditions comes from a variety of areas, such as the visual appearance of the patient, the patient's chief complaint, and the mechanism of injury when trauma is involved. Remember that you should have mastered the components of basic cardiac life support (CPR) before this so that you can draw on that knowledge as you begin to learn how to provide life-saving treatment of immediately and potentially life-threatening conditions. Sometimes, as you begin the initial assessment, you will see something that is obviously abnormal. It may be a cut, a deformed bone, a weakness on one side, abnormal eyes, or some other large abnormality. Avoid being distracted by these conditions; it is easy to let a big cut or deformity draw your attention away from more important, potentially life-threatening problems. By following the steps of the initial assessment you will be able to focus your attention on the condition(s) that may kill a patient, rather than the "grotesque" or obvious injuries that are not necessarily the "life threat".

Table 8-3 (on page 16) lists the components of the initial assessment.

General Impression of the Patient

As you approach the scene and, ultimately, the patient, you will form a general impression of the patient. The general impression is based on your immediate assessment of the environment, the patient's presenting signs and symptoms, and the patient's chief complaint. Examine anything that has a noticeable abnormality.

Priorities of Care

The general impression is important, because it helps you to determine the priorities of care, the mechanism of injury (if trauma was involved), the potential for life-threatening conditions, and the reliability of the information the patient is providing (Figure 8-9).

As you approach the scene, check to see whether the patient is moving or still, awake or unconscious, bleeding or not. Look for the mechanism of injury or the nature of the illness. Listen to what the patient and bystanders have to say. Make note of odors that suggest chemical hazards, smoke, or alcohol on the patient's breath. You can feel for pulses, pain, and deformities when you reach the patient. If the patient is responsive, try to learn as much as possible about what is wrong before you begin your examination. At this time, you should tell the patient your name, identify yourself as an EMT, and explain that you are there to help. You should learn the patient's age, race, gender, and chief complaint and continue to ask questions and talk to a responsive patient throughout the entire assessment.

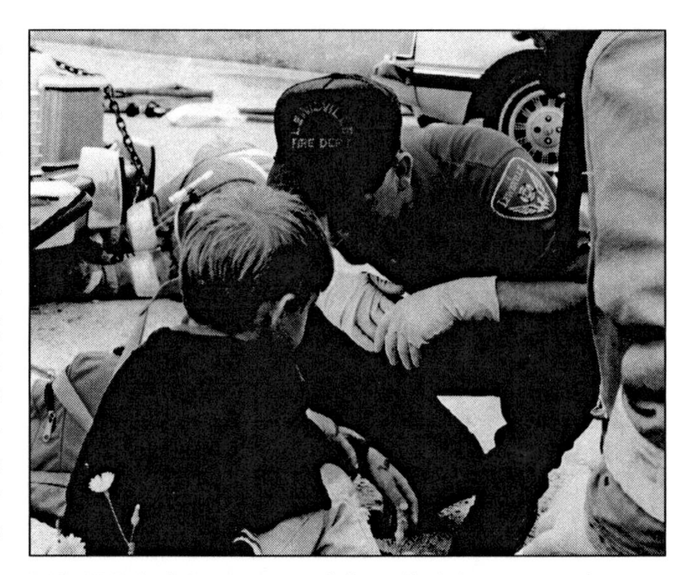

FIGURE 8-9 As you approach the patient, form a general impression of his or her overall condition.

PATIENT ASSESSMENT FLOWCHART

Initial Assessment

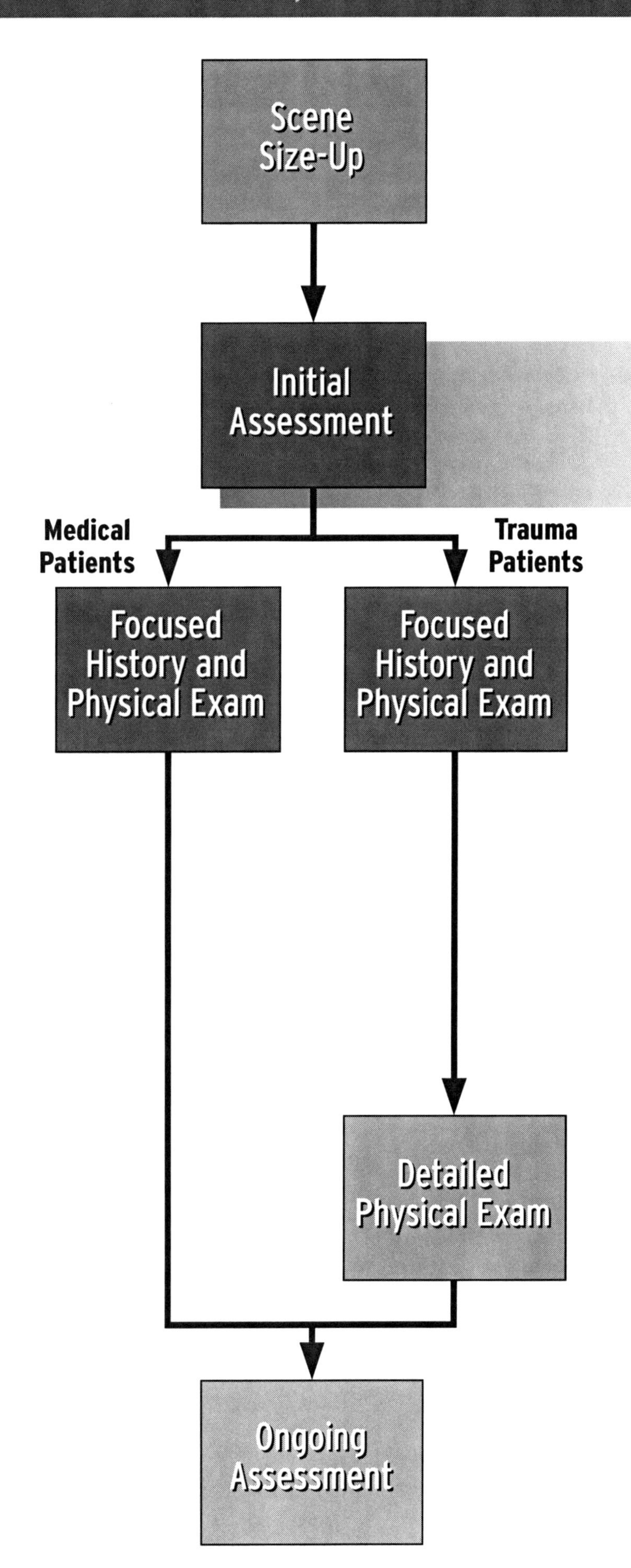

2

TABLE 8-3 Components of the Initial Assessment

Develop a General Impression

- Use the general impression as an overview of the relationship between the mechanism of injury or the nature of the illness, the chief complaint, how the patient looks, and the reliability of the information the patient has given you.
- Assess the patient for a life-threatening condition.

Assess Mental Status (in adults)

- Test for responsiveness:
  Check the patient's response to verbal, tactile, and painful stimuli.
- Test for orientation:
  Check the patient's memory of person, place, time, and event (referred to as alert and oriented times 4).
- Use the AVPU scale to describe patient responsiveness.

Assess Mental Status (in children)

- Determine whether the child is alert:
  Alert infants should track you with their eyes.
  Alert children older than age 2 years should know their own name and that of their parents.
  Alert school-age children should be able to tell you about holidays, school activities, and teachers' names.

Assess Airway

- Responsive patients—Clear airway:
  Talking or crying
- Responsive patients—Partially obstructed airway:
  Noisy breathing (snoring, gurgling, stridor, etc.)
  Speaking only two to three words before each breath
  Retractions or use of accessory muscles
  Nasal flaring (in children)
  Labored breathing

Be prepared to open the airway, administer supplemental oxygen, assist ventilations, and initiate transport procedures.

- Unresponsive patients—Partially obstructed airway:
  Any obvious trauma
  Noisy breathing (snoring, gurgling, stridor, etc.)
  Shallow or absent breathing

Open the airway using the head-tilt/chin-lift or jaw-thrust maneuver.

Assess the Adequacy of Breathing

- Shallow or deep respirations?
- Is the patient choking?
- Is the patient cyanotic?
- Is air moving into and out of the lungs?

If the patient has trouble breathing, make sure the airway is open, and give supplemental oxygen via nonrebreathing mask at 15 L/min. For patients who are breathing at less than 8 breaths/min or more than 24 breaths/min, administer a high concentration of oxygen and consider assisting ventilations if other signs of hypoxia (inadequate oxygenation) are present. Consider a spinal injury in an unresponsive patient who has sustained a traumatic injury, and assist breathing with the proper airway adjunct if the patient is breathing at less than 8 breaths/min or more than 24 breaths/min and also presents with signs of hypoxia.

Assess Circulation

- Assess the quality of the radial pulse.
- Locate and identify any external bleeding.
- Evaluate the skin color, temperature, condition (skin CTC).
- Check capillary refill in patient's less than 6 years old.

Control external bleeding, assist ventilations, and perform CPR (in an unresponsive patient with no pulse) as required. Consider an AED in an unresponsive patient with no obvious traumatic cause of cardiac arrest. Treat the signs and symptoms of hypoperfusion (inadequate circulation).

Identify Priority Patients for Immediate Care and Transport

- Consider:
  Poor general impression
  Unresponsive, with no gag or cough reflexes
  Responsive but unable to follow commands
  Difficulty breathing
  Pale skin/hypoperfusion
  Complicated childbirth
  Uncontrolled bleeding
  Severe pain in any area of the body, disproportionate to the other signs and symptoms presenting.
  Steadily decreasing levels of consciousness
  Severe chest pain, with systolic blood pressure less than 100 mm Hg

Initiate transport as soon as is practical. Consider ALS backup.

You must answer the following questions to begin to form your general impression:

- Does the patient appear to have a life-threatening emergency? Clues could include unconsciousness/unresponsiveness, obvious difficulty breathing and/or noisy breathing, and either cyanotic (blue) or very pale skin color. If you suspect a life-threatening condition, provide immediate care and begin transport procedures.
- Was the patient in an accident? If so, what was the mechanism of injury? On the basis of the mechanism of injury, would you expect the patient to be severely injured? If so, assume the worst and begin treatment, including stabilization of the cervical column.
- Does the patient appear coherent and able to answer questions? If not, you need to rely more heavily on your own assessment skills and/or the information that you can learn from others.

Distinguishing Medical and Trauma Patients

Remember that as a prehospital care provider, you will be called to treat an almost infinite number of different patient problems. Some patients will have a problem that is not related to an accident or trauma; these patients are typically referred to as medical patients. Others will have been injured in an incident such as a fall, a motor vehicle crash, or a shooting. These patients are usually considered trauma patients. In some situations, this distinction will be obvious. If the primary problem appears to be traumatic in origin, you will want to assume the worst and begin treatment, including stabilization of the spinal column. However, quite frequently, it will not. For instance, a patient who falls at a long-term care facility could simply be treated as a trauma patient; however, it is also possible that the fall was caused by a medical condition such as an episode of fainting, a stroke, or even a heart attack. You will learn that it is not always easy or prudent to label patients as medical or trauma until you have finished your assessment. *In many cases, medicine and trauma go hand in hand.*

For this reason, the assessment process does not encourage you to immediately differentiate between medical and trauma patients. Rather, the assessment process begins by assuming that all patients may have both medical and trauma aspects to their condition. Through the assessment process, you will develop an understanding of the patient's problems, both medical and traumatic, and will begin treatment on the basis of that understanding. This approach is both simpler and safer than an approach that starts with an unsupported assumption that the patient is either medical or trauma. As each call unfolds, your patient's primary problem will become apparent.

This rather general assessment is your opportunity to evaluate "the big picture" before you focus on the patient's specific needs, so use all of your senses in observing the scene and patient.

The first steps in caring for any patient focus on finding and treating the most life-threatening illnesses and injuries (Figure 8-10). Through all of these avenues, you need to ask and get answers to the following questions:

- Does the patient have an altered level of consciousness?
- Does the patient have an obstructed airway?
- Does the patient have inadequate breathing?
- Does the patient have inadequate circulation (perfusion)?
- Does the patient have the potential to develop any of these problems?
- Does the patient have the potential for a spinal cord injury?

If the answer to any of these questions is "yes," you need to take immediate action to resolve or prevent the life-threatening condition by doing one of the following: opening the airway, assisting ventilation, giving supplemental oxygen, controlling severe bleeding, performing spinal stabilization, beginning transport procedures, or calling for an ALS unit to assist or assume responsibility for patient care.

Approach to the Assessment Process

Remember, after developing a general impression of the patient, you should begin your assessment and care in this order of importance:

General Impression
Mental Status
Airway
Breathing
Circulation

In all cases, your assessment of the patient's airway, breathing, circulation, (ABC) will govern the extent of treatment performed at the scene. In addition, particularly in the trauma patient, it is important to expose the patient's body completely as soon as possible to facilitate a thorough exam. Always give priority to emergency care of the ABC to ensure life- and limb-saving treatment. Remember to determine the nature of the illness or the mechanism of injury as part of the assessment process.

2

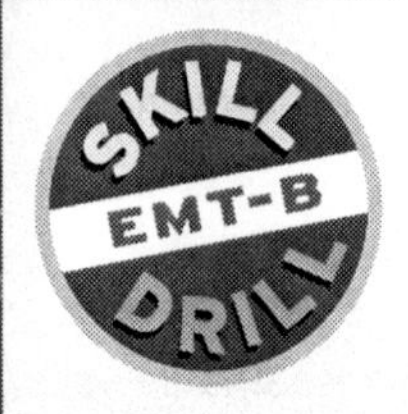

Performing the Initial Assessment

Figure 8-10

2

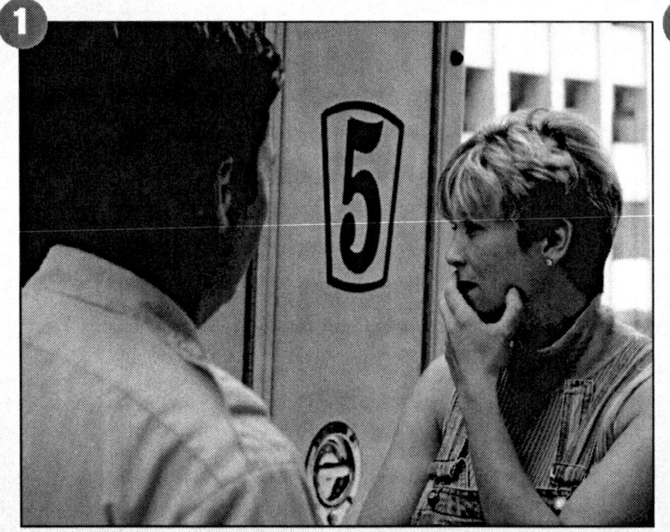

1. Observe the patient to form a general impression.

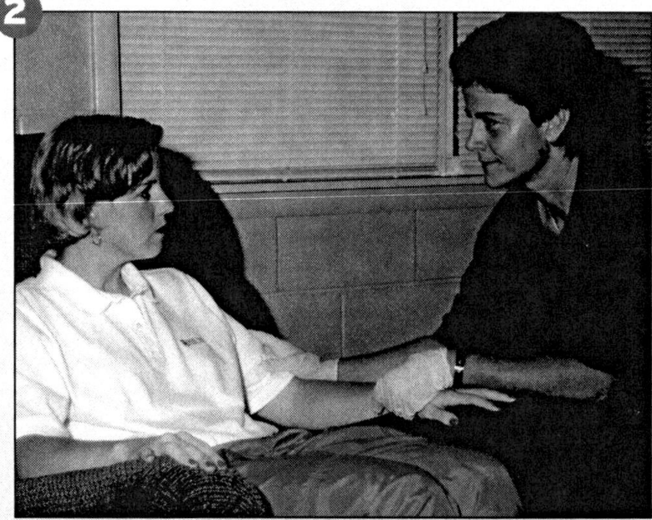

2. Assess the patient's mental status.

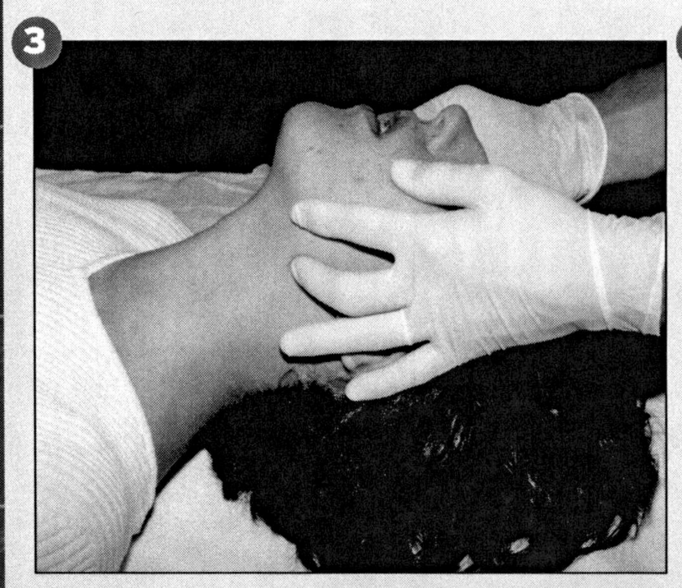

3. To open the airway of a trauma patient use a jaw-thrust or modified jaw-thrust maneuver, both of which cause no movement of the cervical spine. Manual stabilization may also be indicated.

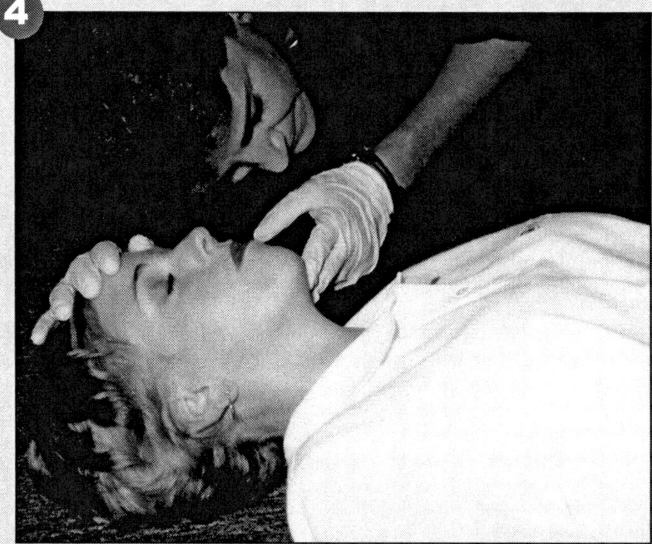

4. Assess breathing using the Look, Listen, and Feel technique. Give supplemental oxygen and/or ventilate if necessary.

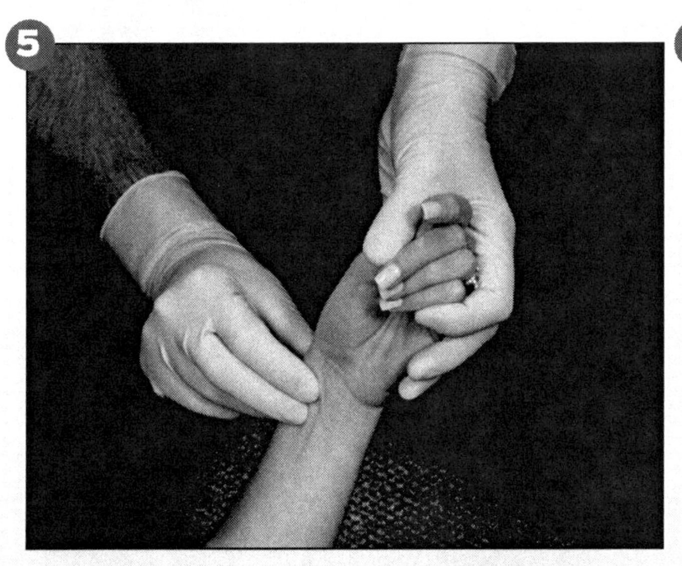

Assess the circulation by taking the pulse, and evaluating skin color, temperature and condition (skin CTC):

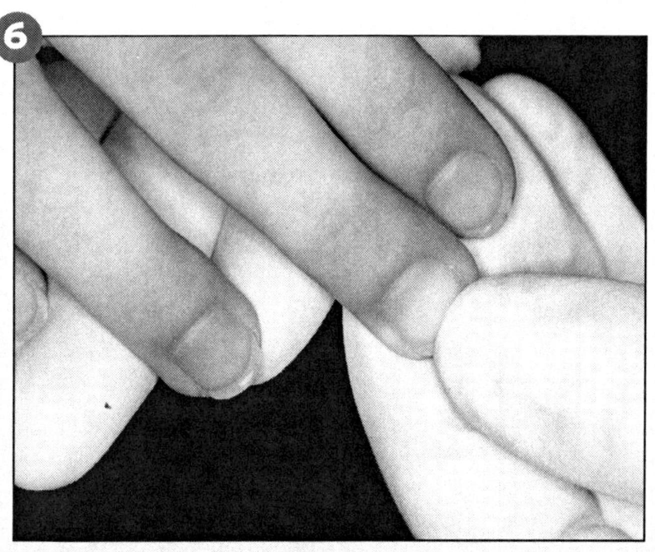

In children, test capillary refill to evaluate circulation (perfusion).

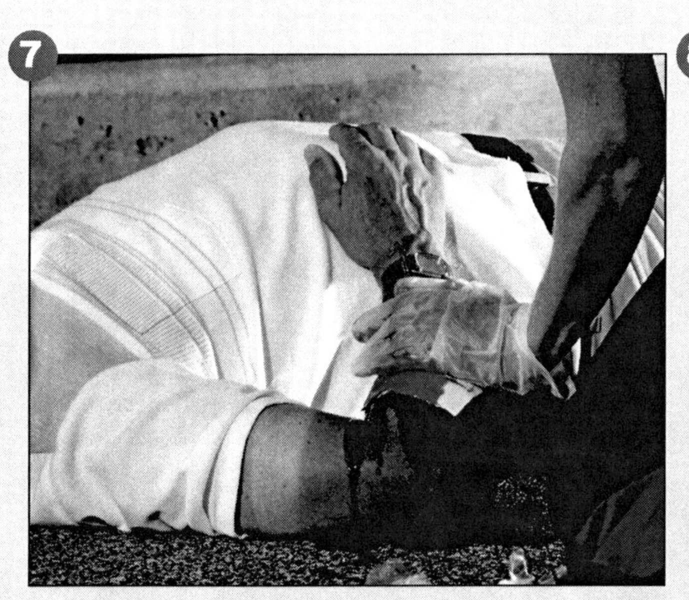

Assess for and control major bleeding.

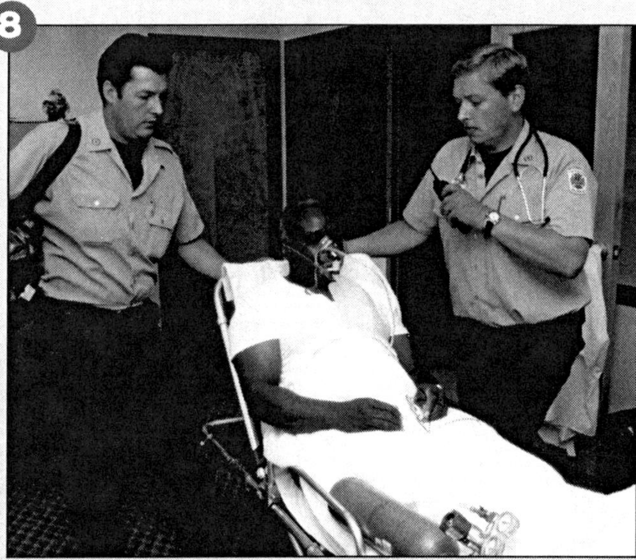

Be prepared to treat life threats and begin transport procedures.

2

communication tip

People call 9-1-1 during some of the most difficult times of their lives. In some cases, they call because of a serious illness or injury. In others, they call because the patient or family is frightened, overwhelmed, or unable to cope with a more minor problem any longer. The patient is often fatigued, sick, frightened, angry, or sad, and the family often shares some or all of these feelings. Regardless of the exact nature of the call, the patient, family, and bystanders expect you to bring comfort, control, and resolution of these problems—emotional and physical.

In many ways, good communication skills are as important as technical proficiency, if not more so. Each step in the assessment process can be impeded by poor communication, and each can be immeasurably benefited by a good connection between you and the patient and family. Here are five tips that can vastly improve your communication skills during the assessment process:

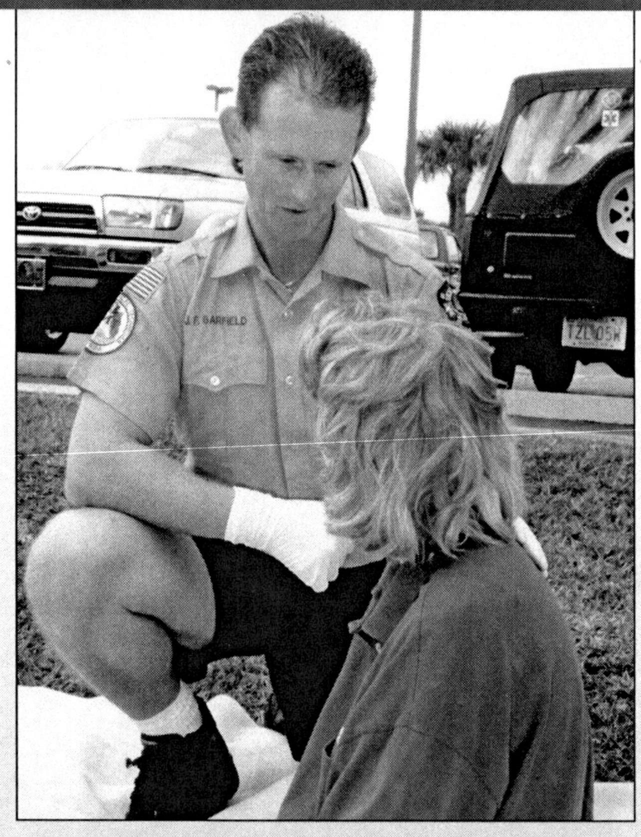

FIGURE 8-11 Position yourself near the patient, at eye level when possible, to begin to establish a relationship with the patient.

1. **Do whatever you can, quickly, to make yourself and the patient comfortable.** Patients are uncomfortable communicating with someone who is standing over them, pacing, or looking away. When time permits, sit down and/or position yourself near the patient, introduce yourself, and ask the patient's name (Figure 8-11). This simple action signals the patient that you have time to talk; it opens the channels of communication as nothing else will. At the same time, be conscious of the patient's personal space. Do not move in too quickly. Ask the patient whether there is something you can do to make him or her more comfortable. Caring gestures and good body language are a visible demonstration of your care and concern.

Assessing Mental Status

Evaluating a patient's mental status and level of consciousness is an important part of the initial assessment because the mental status reflects the functioning of the brain. Remember to maintain spinal stabilization if needed. Many conditions may alter brain function and hence the level of consciousness. You will learn about many of these conditions as you progress through the EMT-B course.

Mental status and level of consciousness can be evaluated in just a few seconds by using two separate tests: responsiveness and orientation. The test for responsiveness assesses how well a patient responds to external stimuli, including verbal stimuli (sound), and tactile stimuli (touch). For a patient who is alert and responding to verbal stimuli, you should next evaluate orientation. Orientation tests assess mental status by checking the patient's memory of person (his or her name), place (the current location), time (the current year, month, time of day, and approximate date), and event (what happened). These four questions were not selected at random. They evaluate long-term memory (name and place if the patient is at home), intermediate-term memory (place and time), and short-term memory (event). If the patient knows these facts, the patient is said to be "alert and oriented times four" ("times four" refers to person, place, time, and event). An example of a patient who is not fully oriented would be one who is "alert and oriented times two, disoriented to time and event." Loss of intermediate- and long-term memory (person and place) is thought to

2. **Actively listen to the patient.** In many cases, patients will be able to tell you what is wrong with them if you are paying attention and are truly listening. You can use several skills to actively listen, including leaning in toward the patient, taking selective notes, and periodically repeating back important points to the patient to ensure that you understood correctly. Active listening is often more difficult than it might seem, because scenes are often noisy and chaotic, and you will be receiving information from the patient, the family, your partner, and other EMS, fire, or law enforcement individuals on the scene. Try to screen them out for a few minutes so that you can truly listen to the patient; it will pay big dividends.
3. **Make eye contact with the person with whom you are speaking.** Eye contact signals that you are listening, so the patient is more likely to open up. An added benefit is that you will see facial expressions that, in some cases, communicate more clearly than the patient's words. For instance, you might see a facial grimace of pain or the averted eyes indicating embarrassment. Note that some cultures are uncomfortable with or offended by direct eye contact. Be sure to be familiar with the customs of people in your area.
4. **Base your initial questions on the patient's complaints.** No one likes to think that he or she is "just another patient." But that is what you communicate if you always ask the same questions of every patient, regardless of their complaints. If you ask questions about their Medicare number while they are trying to tell you about their pain, you are communicating that you are not really interested in their problem. Talk about their problem first, then ask paperwork questions.
5. **Before you start treatment, stop for a moment and mentally summarize what you have learned and what you are going to do, then tell the patient.** By providing necessary information to the patient and family, you help to relieve their anxiety and fear. This will also give them an opportunity to give you additional information if you have missed something.

You should spend your entire EMS career fine-tuning your patient assessment skills, as they are the cornerstone of high-quality prehospital care. A poor assessment almost always results in substandard patient care. Be sure to focus some of your energy on improving the communication process. You will make it easier for patients to feel comfortable around you, which will help them to give honest, direct answers to your questions. As a result, you will get better assessment information in less time.

be related to more severe problems than loss of short-term memory. Collectively, your evaluation of the patient's responsiveness and orientation will paint a picture of the overall mental status.

Responsiveness can be evaluated by using the AVPU scale:

- **Alert.** The patient's eyes open spontaneously as you approach, and the patient appears aware of and responsive to the environment. The patient appears to follow commands, and the eyes visually track people and objects.
- **Responsive to Verbal Stimulus.** The patient's eyes do not open spontaneously. However, the patient's eyes do open to verbal stimuli, and the patient is able to respond in some meaningful way when spoken to.

caring for kids

Mental status may be difficult to evaluate in children. First, determine whether the child is alert. Even infants should be alert to your presence and should follow you with their eyes (a process called "tracking"). Ask the parent whether the child is behaving normally, particularly as regards alertness. All children older than age 2 years should know their own name and the names of their parents and siblings. Evaluate mental status in school-age children by asking about holidays, recent school activities, or teacher's names.

2

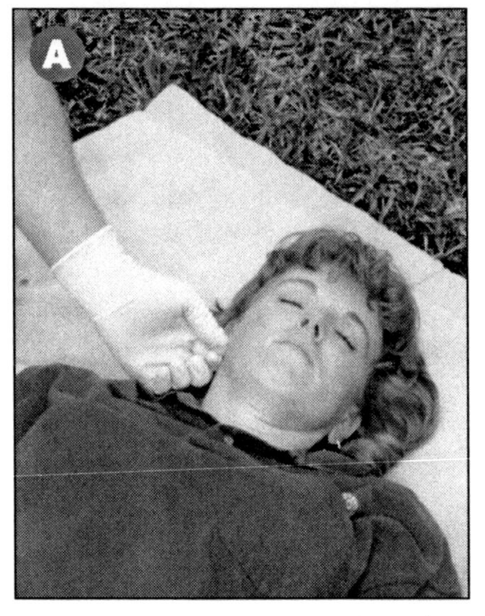

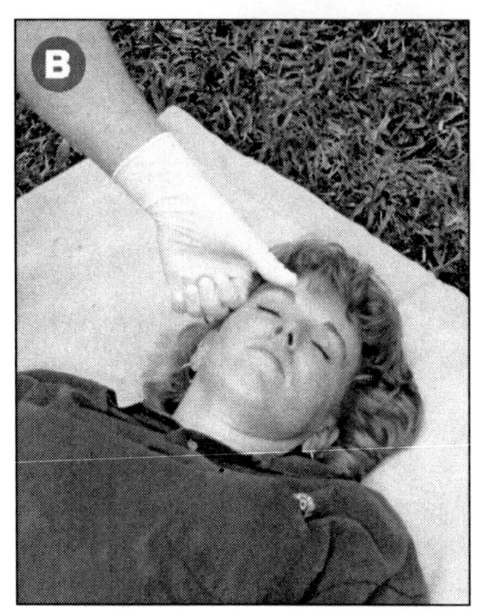

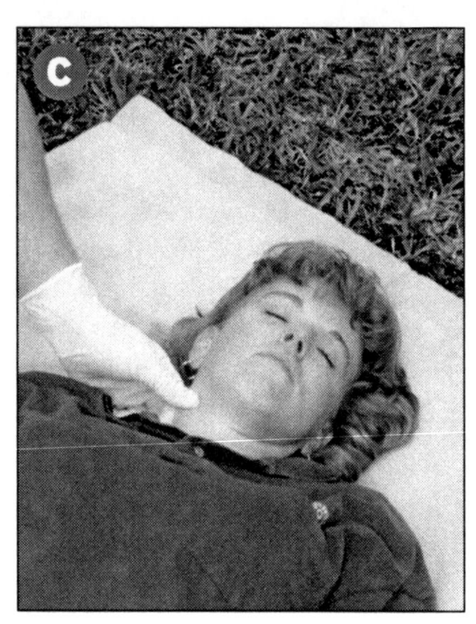

FIGURE 8-12 **A:** Gently but firmly pinch the patient's earlobe. **B:** Press down on the bone above the eye. **C:** Pinch the muscles of the neck.

- **Responsive to Pain.** The patient does not respond to your questions but moves or cries out in response to a painful stimulus. This response is tested by gently but firmly pinching the patient's earlobe, by pressing down on the bone above the eye, or by pinching the muscles of the neck (Figure 8-12). An appropriate response is moaning or pushing away or withdrawing from the pinch. Use of extremely painful stimuli is never appropriate. The sternal rub, although advocated in CPR training, is not recommended because it may be inaccurate in patients with cervical spine injuries. The use of ammonia "smelling salts" is also not recommended.
- **Unresponsive.** The patient does not respond to any stimuli.

If you are in doubt about whether a patient is truly unconscious, assume the worst and treat appropriately.

An abnormal mental status may be caused by a wide variety of conditions, including head trauma, hypoxia (inadequate oxygenation), hypoglycemia (low blood sugar), stroke, cardiac problems, or drug use. If the patient has an abnormal mental status, you should rapidly complete the initial assessment and be prepared to give high-flow supplemental oxygen, consider spinal stabilization if trauma is suspected, and initiate transport procedures. Support the ABC as required, and continually reassess for changes in the patient's condition.

Airway obstruction in an unconscious patient is most commonly due to relaxation of the tongue muscles back into throat.

Assessing the Airway

As you move through the steps of assessment, you must always be alert for signs of respiratory compromise or airway obstruction. Regardless of the cause, airway obstruction may result in inadequate or absent air flow into and out of the lungs, which may cause permanent damage to the brain, heart, and lungs or may even result in death.

Responsive Patients

Patients of any age who are responsive and are talking or crying have an open airway. However, watching and listening to how patients speak, particularly those with respiratory problems, may provide important clues about the adequacy of their airway and breathing status.

If you identify an airway problem, stop the assessment process, and open the airway using the head-tilt/chin-lift or jaw-thrust maneuver. Although airway and breathing problems are not the same, their signs and symptoms often overlap. A patient who can speak only two to three words without pausing to take a breath, a condition known as two- to three-word dyspnea, has a severe airway obstruction (a narrowing of the airways caused by trauma or disease) or other breathing problem. The presence of retractions or the use of the accessory muscles of respiration is also a sign of airway obstruction. Nasal flaring and use of the accessory muscles indicate that a child has an airway obstruction. Finally, obviously labored breathing is also a sign of airway or breathing difficulties.

Any of these signs may signal an immediate or pending airway and/or breathing problem. You should be prepared to open the airway, administer supplemental oxygen, assist ventilation, and initiate transport procedures.

Unresponsive Patients

With an unresponsive patient or one with diminished responsiveness, you should immediately assess the patency of the airway. If it is clear, you can continue your assessment. If the airway is not clear, your next priority is to open it using the head-tilt/chin-lift or jaw-thrust maneuver. Airway obstruction in an unconscious patient is most commonly due to relaxation of the tongue muscles back into throat. Dentures, blood clots, vomitus, mucus, food, or other foreign objects may also create a blockage. Signs of airway obstruction in an unconscious patient include the following:

- Obvious trauma, blood, or other obstruction
- Noisy breathing, such as snoring, bubbling, gurgling, crowing, or other abnormal sounds (Normal breathing is quiet.)
- Extremely shallow or absent breathing (Airway obstruction may cause impaired breathing.)

To open the airway, positioning depends on the patient's age and size. For medical patients, perform the head-tilt/chin-lift maneuver. For trauma patients or those with illness of an unknown nature, the cervical spine should be manually stabilized, and, if necessary, the jaw-thrust maneuver should be performed.

Assessing Breathing

As you assess the patient's breathing, look at how much work it takes for the patient to breathe. Normal respirations are not unusually shallow or excessively deep, and their rate varies widely in adults, anywhere from 12 to 20 breaths/min. Shallow respirations can be identified by minimal movement of the chest wall. Conversely, deep respirations cause a great deal of chest wall rise and fall and often can be heard as large volumes of air moving into and out of the patient's lungs. As you assess the patient, ask yourself the following questions:

- Are the patient's respirations shallow or deep?
- Does the patient appear to be choking?
- Is the patient cyanotic (blue)?
- Is the patient moving air into and out of the lungs as the chest rises and falls?

If a patient seems to have difficulty breathing, you should immediately reevaluate the airway. Once the airway is open, determine if breathing is adequate. You should *consider* assisting ventilation with a BVM device if the patient presents with signs and symptoms of hypoxia *and* respirations are greater than 24/min or less than 8/min.

Any patient with a decreased level of consciousness, respiratory distress, or poor skin color should, at least, receive high-flow oxygen. If there is no risk of spinal cord injury, the patient should remain in a comfortable position that supports breathing; this is typically sitting up with the legs dangling. In any patient who has a possible risk for spinal injury, you should stabilize the spine, ensuring that respirations are not compromised while you restrict spinal motion.

You should give supplemental oxygen via a nonrebreathing mask at 15 L/min. Any patient whom you identify as having immediate or potential airway or breathing problems should be given supplemental oxygen. Never withhold oxygen from any patient at the scene!

Use the Look, Listen, and Feel technique to evaluate how well an unconscious patient is breathing. This technique is equally effective in most patients, although it may be more difficult in infants and small children because they have so little chest wall movement during respirations. If the patient does not appear to be breathing or has a compromised airway, start airway management immediately, and assist ventilation.

In most cases, a spinal injury should be considered a possibility for any unresponsive trauma patient. These patients must be rolled or moved as a single unit onto a flat surface or backboard. The timing for this maneuver depends on the patient's position when you find him or her. If the patient must be moved to access the face or manage the airway, it should be done immediately. Otherwise, you should log roll the patient after you attend to ABC. Remember, you must move the head, neck, torso, and legs as a unit without any unnecessary bending or twisting.

Once the patient is properly positioned and the airway is opened, you may begin to support the patient's breathing. If the patient presents with obvious signs and symptoms of hypoxia *and* respirations of 24/min or more, or 8/min or less, you should consider ventilating with the proper airway adjuncts.

If the patient is not breathing, open and maintain the airway and provide rescue breathing using the appropriate airway adjuncts. Whenever you use the BVM device, supplemental oxygen should be provided as well.

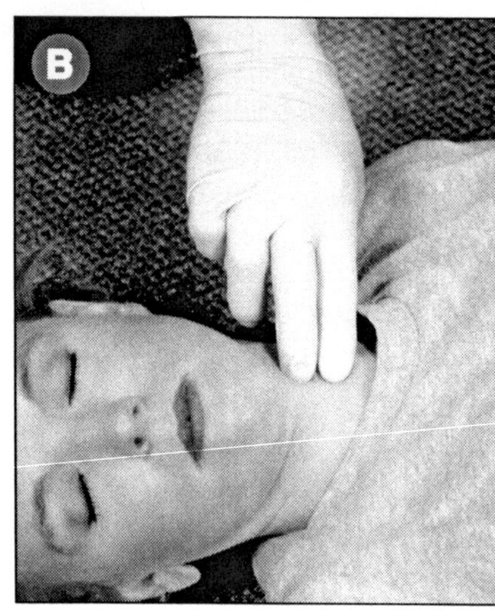

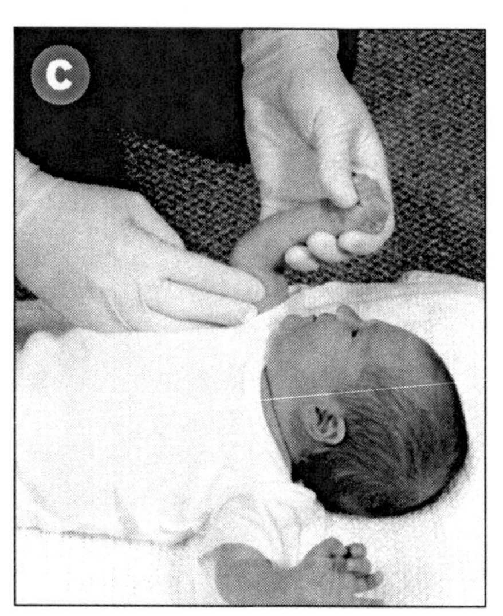

FIGURE 8-13 **A:** Palpate the radial artery to initially evaluate the pulse. **B:** Palpate the carotid artery if you cannot feel a pulse at the radial artery. **C:** In infants palpate the brachial artery to evaluate the pulse.

Assessing Circulation

Assessing circulation helps you to evaluate how well blood is circulating to the major organs, including the brain, lungs, heart, kidneys, and rest of the body. A variety of problems can impair circulation, including blood loss, conditions that affect the heart, and conditions that affect the major blood vessels. Circulation is evaluated by assessing the presence and qualities of the pulse, identifying the presence of serious external bleeding, and evaluating skin color, temperature, and condition (skin CTC).

If the patient does not have a radial pulse, check for a carotid pulse. If the patient has a carotid pulse but is still not breathing, continue rescue breathing at a rate of 12 to 20 breaths/min for an adult, or 20 to 25 breaths/min for a child, until the patient begins breathing adequately again. You should continuously assess the pulse to determine whether rescue breathing has been effective in an unresponsive patient. When rescue breathing is not done properly, the pulse will stop, and the patient will go into cardiac arrest. If this occurs, you should begin CPR immediately.

Assessing the Pulse

The rate, rhythm, and strength of the patient's pulse will give you a rough idea of the overall status of the patient's cardiac function. The pulse is one of the vital signs that you should monitor continuously in most patients, even enroute to the hospital.Pulse rate is measured by palpating (feeling) an artery at a pulse point, which is an area where an artery lies close to the surface of the skin (Figure 8-13) and is expressed in terms of beats per minute. As you evaluate the pulse, note whether it is strong or weak and whether it is regular or irregular. For an alert, responsive patient, the contact from your hands taking the pulse can be a very reassuring gesture.

The most common place to palpate (examine by touch) for the pulse in an adult patient is at the wrist, along the radial artery. If you cannot feel a pulse at either wrist, you should try to find it in the neck at the carotid artery. The carotid pulse is easier to locate than the radial pulse, especially if the patient has falling blood pressure. The carotid pulse is most easily located by first finding the patient's Adam's apple at the front of the neck. You should then slide your index and middle fingers along one side of the neck until you feel the pulse. The carotid pulse can be felt along a groove between the larynx (voice box) and one of the neck muscles. In an unresponsive patient, you should palpate the carotid pulse first. Although the normal pulse rate varies depending upon the patient's underlying physical conditions, most sources suggest that a pulse rate of 60 to 100 beats/min is normal in adults.

If you do not find a pulse, even at the carotid artery, you must take immediate action. For a medical patient over 8 years old or greater than 55 lb, start CPR and apply an AED. For a medical patient under 8 or who weighs less than 55 lb, start CPR without using the AED. For a trauma patient of any age in cardiac arrest, start CPR.

Assessing and Controlling External Bleeding

The next step is to identify any major external bleeding. In some instances, blood loss can be very rapid and can quickly result in shock (inadequate perfusion) and even

caring for kids

You can feel the pulse of a child at the carotid artery, as in an adult. However, palpating this pulse in an infant may present a problem. Because an infant's neck is often very short and fat, and its pulse is often quite fast, you may have a hard time finding the carotid pulse. Therefore, in infants younger than one year of age, you should palpate the brachial artery to assess the pulse. Normal pulse rates for children are shown in Table 8-4.

TABLE 8-4 Normal Pulse Rates in Infants and Children

Age	Range
Newborn	120 to 160
Infant	120 to 140
1 to 3 years	100 to 110
3 to 5 years	90 to 100
5 to 10 years	80 to 100
10 to 15 years	60 to 90
Over 15 years	Adult normal ranges

death. Therefore, this step demands your immediate attention as soon as the patient's airway is secured and breathing is stabilized. Signs of blood loss include active bleeding from wounds and/or evidence of bleeding such as blood on the clothes or near the patient. Serious bleeding from a large vein may be characterized by steady blood flow. Bleeding from an artery is characterized by a spurting flow of blood. When you evaluate an unconscious patient, do a sweep for blood by quickly and lightly running your gloved hands from head to toe, pausing periodically to see whether your gloves are bloody.

Controlling external bleeding is often very simple. In almost all instances, direct pressure with your gloved hand and a sterile bandage over the bleeding site will control bleeding. This pressure stops the flow of blood and helps the blood to coagulate, or clot naturally. Remember that you must follow BSI techniques whenever you may be exposed to blood or other body fluids.

Most often, bleeding can be adequately controlled by using direct pressure over the bleeding site, along with elevating the extremity if bleeding is on the arms or legs. When direct pressure and elevation are not successful, you may apply pressure directly over arterial pressure points. Another option to control bleeding is use of the pneumatic antishock garment (PASG) for widespread bleeding over the legs and/or pelvic region. However, there are a number of precautions regarding the PASG; including local protocol; these, along with specific information on bleeding control, are described in Chapters 24 and 25 on bleeding and shock.

Evaluating Skin Color, Temperature, and Condition

Assessing the skin is one of the most important and most readily accessible ways of evaluating circulation (perfusion). You should assess the patient's skin color, temperature, and condition (skin CTC), as well as look for bleeding.

Color. Skin color depends on pigmentation and blood oxygen levels, as well as the amount of blood circulating through the vessels of the skin. For this reason, skin color is a valuable assessment tool. The normal skin color of lightly pigmented people is pinkish. Deeply pigmented skin may hide color changes that result from illness or injury. Therefore, you should look for changes in color in areas of the skin that have less pigment: the fingernail beds (assess peripheral perfusion), the sclera (white of the eyes), the conjunctiva (lining of the eyelid), and the mucous membranes of the mouth (assess central perfusion). Normal skin color, particularly of the conjunctivae and mucous membranes, is pinkish. Skin colors that should alert you to possible medical problems include cyanosis (blue), flushed (red), pale (lack of color), and jaundice (yellow).

Temperature. The skin is actually an organ, and like all other organs, it has many functions. It helps maintain the water content of the body, acts as insulation and

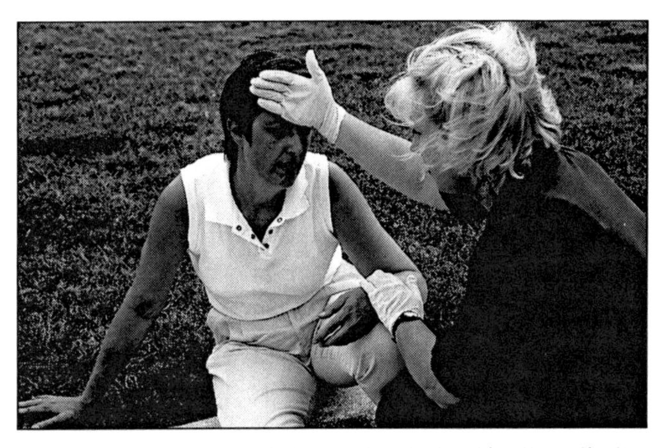

FIGURE 8-14 Assess skin temperature by touching the patient's skin with the back of your gloved hand.

2

> When rescue breathing is not done properly, the pulse will stop, and the patient will go into cardiac arrest.

protection from infection, and also plays a role in regulation of body temperature. Normal body temperature is 98.6°F (37°C), but it can change as a result of illness or injury. Assess the skin temperature by touching the patient's skin with your gloved hand (Figure 8-14).

Condition. Finally, determine whether the patient's skin is dry or moist. The skin is normally warm and dry. Cool or cold, moist, clammy skin suggests shock (inadequate perfusion). Hot skin may indicate an abnormally elevated body temperature.

Evaluating capillary refill. Another way to assess circulation is to check capillary refill, especially in infants and children less than 6 years old. Capillary refill is the ability of the circulatory system to return blood to the capillaries after circulation has been interrupted. You test capillary refill by squeezing the patient's fingernail bed until the area blanches (turns white) (Figure 8-15). Next release the fingernail bed, and watch for it to return to a normal color. The area should return to its normal color within two seconds. If the area remains white or becomes blue, you know that circulation is inadequate, at least in the area being tested.

Capillary refill can be checked in children by squeezing the entire arm or leg at a distal point and observing the return to normal color. Although capillary refill is a quick and very general way to evaluate circulation, it is important to remember that other conditions, not related to the circulatory system, may also slow capillary refill. These conditions include the patient's age and gender, as well as exposure to a cold environment (hypothermia), frozen tissue (frostbite), or injuries to bones or muscles that cause local circulatory compromise (i.e., a fracture of the radius causing loss of distal circulation).

Restoring circulation. If a patient has inadequate circulation, you must take immediate action to restore or improve circulation, control severe bleeding if present, and improve oxygen delivery to the tissues. The *absence* of a distal palpable pulse in a *responsive* patient is not caused by cardiac arrest. Therefore, do not begin CPR in a responsive patient. However, if you cannot feel a carotid pulse in an unresponsive adult patient, you should immediately begin CPR and, whenever possible and indicated, prepare to defibrillate. Remember to follow BSI techniques, which may include use of a barrier device for ventilation, gloves, and perhaps goggles. Follow these five steps in a patient who has no pulse and is unresponsive:

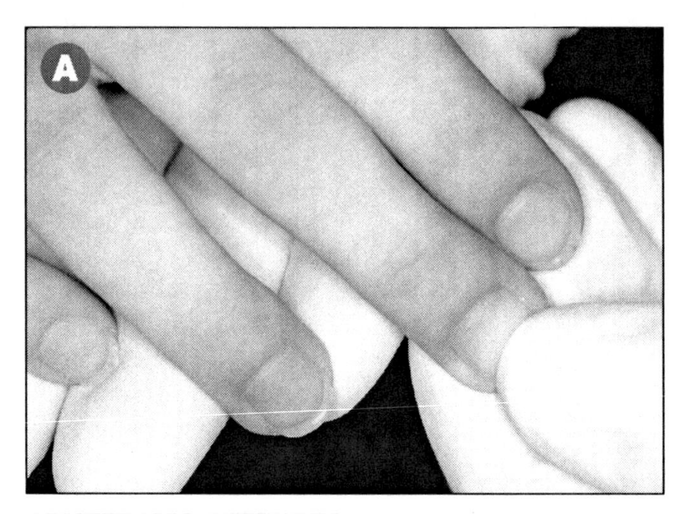

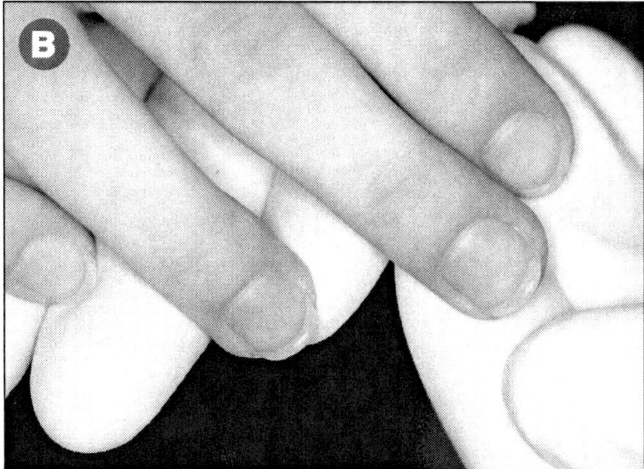

FIGURE 8-15 **A:** Test capillary refill by squeezing the patient's fingernail bed until the area blanches. **B:** Release the fingernail and watch for it to return to its normal color.

1. **Immediately begin CPR** if no automated external defibrillator (AED) is available. If an AED is readily available, apply it first, following local protocol.
2. **Prepare to use the AED** if the patient is older than 8 years of age or weighs more than 55 lb and has no obvious traumatic cause of cardiac arrest. Local protocols may vary on the age and weight requirements for AED use.

3. **If the cardiac arrest is associated** with an obvious, apparently catastrophic traumatic event, perform CPR without use of the AED. Traumatic arrests do not typically respond to defibrillation, particularly since the majority of traumatic arrests are caused by severe blood loss (hypovolemia). Attempting to use the AED on a victim of hypovolemia would be comparable to trying to jump start a car that ran out of gas. Treatment of traumatic arrest should include initiation of airway control, ventilation, and chest compressions, followed by transport to the hospital. Immediate transport to the hospital, preferably a trauma center, is the most valuable therapy for the patient in traumatic cardiac arrest.
4. **Initiate use of the AED** in association with CPR, if in doubt about a traumatic origin of the arrest or if local protocol indicates the use as appropriate (i.e. electrocution or drownings).
5. **Prepare for rapid transport** to an appropriate facility.

Continued impaired circulation is devastating to the body's cells because it denies them vital oxygen, which is necessary for cell function. CPR and bleeding control are intended to maintain or improve circulation. Oxygen delivery is improved through the administration of supplemental oxygen. Any patient with impaired circulation (inadequate perfusion) should receive high-flow oxygen via a non-rebreathing mask or assisted ventilations to improve oxygen delivery at the cellular level.

Identifying Priority Patients

To complete the initial assessment, you have to make some decisions about patient care. You should have already addressed life-threatening injuries and/or illnesses as they are found. Next, you must identify priority patients, or those who need other interventions and/or rapid transport.

Patients with one of the following conditions should be given priority care and/or rapid transport or be considered for ALS backup:

- Poor general impression
- Unresponsive with no gag or cough reflexes
- Responsive but unable to follow commands
- Difficulty breathing
- Pale skin or other signs of poor perfusion
- Complicated childbirth
- Uncontrolled bleeding
- Severe pain (disproportionate to the other signs and symptoms that present)
- Severe chest pain, especially when the systolic blood pressure is less than 100 mm Hg

Correct identification of high-priority patients is an essential aspect of the initial assessment and helps to improve patient outcome.

While life-saving treatment is important, it is essential to remember that rapid transport is one of the keys to the survival of any high priority patient. Transport procedures should be initiated as soon as is practical and possible for high priority patients.

Once you complete the steps of the initial assessment, which include the general impression, mental status, airway, breathing, circulation, and identification of priority patients, you then proceed to the appropriate focused history and physical exam based on your current assessment of whether the patient you are treating has problems of traumatic origin, medical origin, or both.

2

Focused History and Physical Exam: Trauma Patients

You now have dispatch information and information from both the scene size-up and initial assessment. These have provided you with valuable information about the scene, allowing you to anticipate what you will find and prepare for hazards. If your patient had problems with ABC, you have stabilized any life-threatening conditions, perhaps provided spinal stabilization, and initiated transport procedures.

How do you proceed now? Your patient may have, almost literally, one or more of a million different problems. How do you identify, prioritize, and treat this variety of potential problems?

Goals of the Focused History and Physical Exam

The focused history and physical exam help you to focus on specific problems. The goals of the focused history and physical exam are:

1. Understand the specific circumstances surrounding the chief complaint.
   - What circumstances were associated with the event?
   - Is the mechanism of injury a high risk for serious injuries?
   - Has this happened before? What were the cause and treatment then?
2. Direct further physical examination.
   - What additional problems can be identified through the physical exam?

The focused history and physical exam, like the entire assessment process, guide you to take actions that will stabilize or relieve the patient's problems. Depending on the answers to the questions and exams performed here, you should be prepared to return to the initial assessment if potentially life-threatening conditions are identified. The focused history and physical exam: trauma is performed after the initial assessment and includes the physical exam, baseline vital signs and history. The steps of the focused history and physical exam are altered based on how the patient presents. If there is a mechanism of injury, you will perform the focused history and physical exam for the trauma patient. When the patient has a complaint that is medical in nature, and you have confirmed that there is no mechanism of injury, you will perform the focused history and physical exam for the medical patient.

As part of the focused history and physical exam: trauma, be prepared to perform spinal immobilization if indicated, provide transport or coordinate transfer of the patient to an ALS unit, and/or treat any problems that you identify during the exam.

Patients who call 9-1-1 following a sudden event may have any number of problems—medical, traumatic, or a combination of both. Unfortunately, patients do not wear signs identifying them as "medical" or "trauma." Furthermore, the circumstances surrounding the event may ultimately identify medical causes of trauma or traumatic problems that worsened a medical condition. For this reason, to consider any patient strictly as "medical" or "trauma" can be difficult and sometimes inaccurate. Rather, you should begin an assessment and manage all patients in the same systematic fashion. However, as each case unfolds, it will often become apparent that the patient's problem is predominantly traumatic or medical in nature. When this occurs, you should focus your assessment on the medical or traumatic aspects of the case.

Once you have identified that a patient has sustained a traumatic injury, you need to rapidly make some important treatment and transport decisions. This is because some traumatic injuries are life-threatening and cannot be treated in the field. High priority trauma patients have the best chance for survival if they arrive

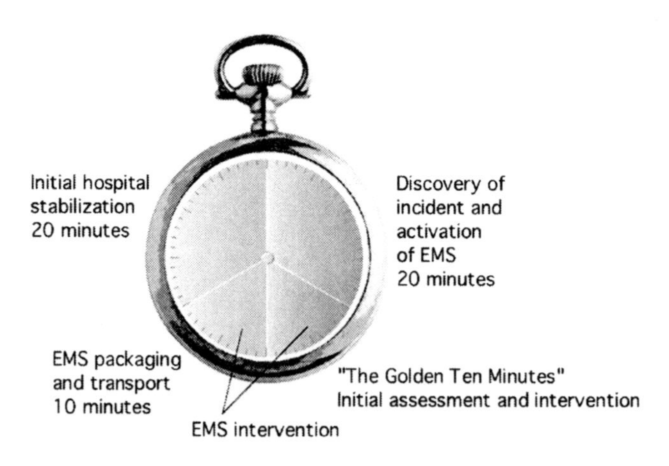

FIGURE 8-16 The Golden Hour is the time during which treatment of shock (inadequate perfusion) or traumatic injuries is most critical and the potential for survival is best.

PATIENT ASSESSMENT FLOWCHART

Focused History and Physical Exam: Trauma Patients

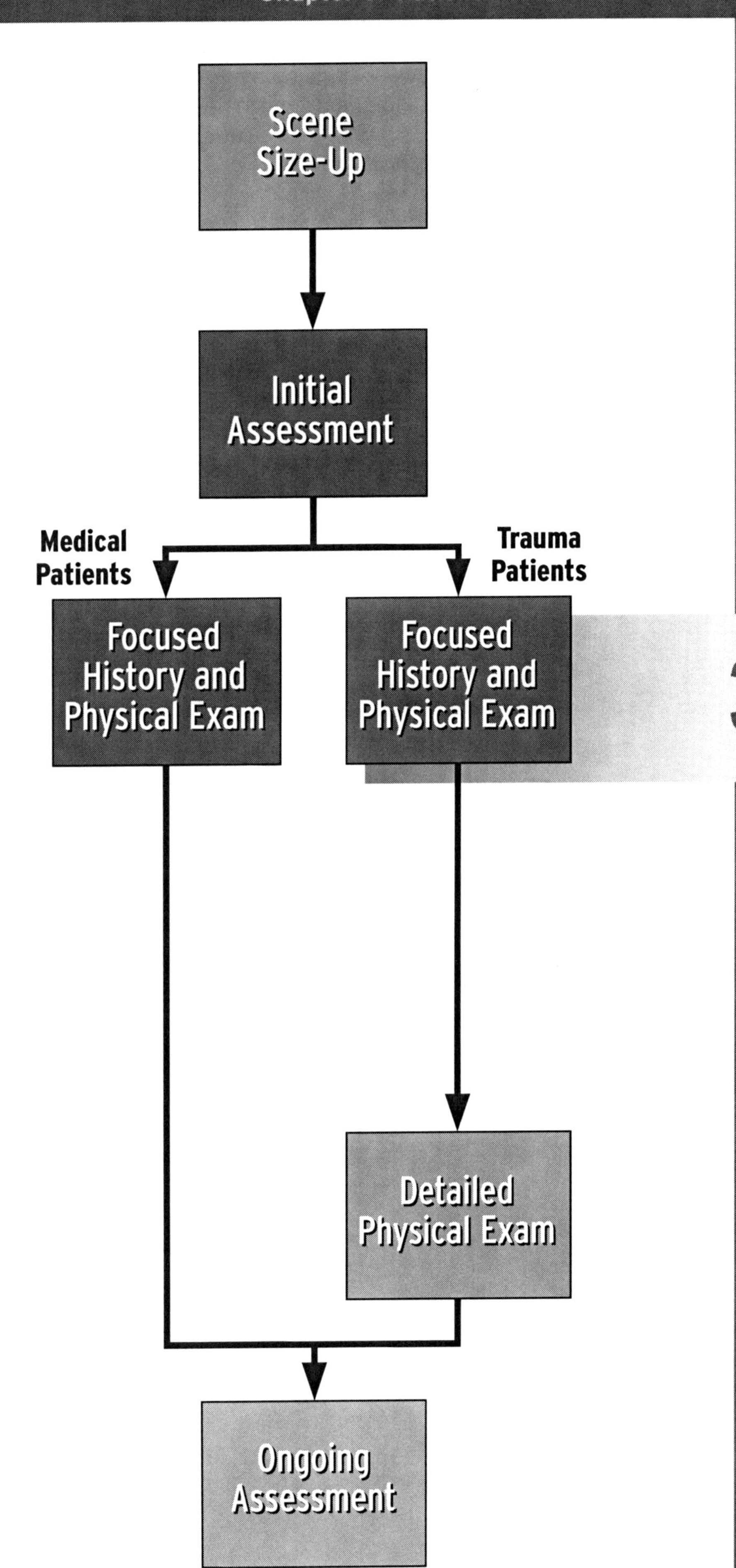

3

at an appropriate hospital, usually a trauma center if available, for definitive care. Definitive care describes treatment provided to cure or resolve a patient's current illness or injury (i.e. surgery to repair a badly fractured leg or uncontrollable bleed). *Ideally*, definitive care should occur within 60 minutes of the time of injury. You will often hear this time period called the Golden Hour. The Golden Hour is the time during which treatment of shock (inadequate perfusion) or traumatic injuries is most critical and survival potential is the best (Figure 8-16). After the first 60 minutes, the body has increasing difficulty in compensating for traumatic injuries.

For this reason, you should spend as little of the Golden Hour as possible on the scene with patients who have suffered significant mechanism of injury or severe trauma. Table 8-5 lists the components of the focused history and physical exam for the trauma patient.

TABLE 8-5 Components of the Focused History and Physical Exam: Trauma Patient

Significant Mechanism of Injury

- Ejection from a vehicle
- A death in the passenger compartment
- A fall greater than 20' (greater than 10' for children)
- Vehicle rollover
- High-speed vehicle collision
- Medium-speed vehicle collision (for children)
- Vehicle-pedestrian collision
- Motorcycle accident
- Bicycle collision (for children)
- Unresponsiveness or altered mental status
- Hidden injuries from seat belts, airbags, etc.

Reconsider the Mechanism of Injury (MOI)

- Perform a rapid trauma assessment (on either a responsive or unresponsive patient who has suffered a significant MOI).
- Take a baseline set of vital signs.
- Obtain a SAMPLE history.

No Significant Mechanism of Injury

- Assess the chief complaint.
- Perform a focused trauma assessment.
- Take a baseline set of vital signs.
- Obtain a SAMPLE history.

Reconsider the Mechanism of Injury

As part of the scene size-up, you evaluated the mechanism of injury before you began treatment. During the focused history and physical exam: trauma, you should look at the mechanism again to ensure that you have not missed important information. Awareness of the mechanism of injury helps you to understand the severity, or potential severity, of the patient's problem, as well as, provide invaluable information to hospital staff. Some patients have experienced a significant mechanism of injury; others clearly have not.

Significant Mechanisms of Injury

Significant mechanisms of injury include the following:

- Ejection from a vehicle
- A death in the same passenger compartment
- Fall greater than 20'
- Vehicle rollover
- High-speed vehicle collision
- Vehicle-pedestrian collision
- Motorcycle crash
- Unresponsiveness or altered mental status
- Penetrating head, chest, or abdominal trauma
- Hidden injuries from seat belts, airbags, etc.

Infant and Child Considerations

Significant mechanisms of injury for children include the above with the following additions or modifications:

- Fall greater than 10'
- Bicycle crash
- Medium-speed vehicle collision

Hidden Injuries

Seat belts and airbags have significantly reduced the death and disability that are associated with motor vehicle accidents. However, you should be aware that seat belts and airbags can also cause injuries. When evaluating a patient who was involved in a motor vehicle crash, you should ask questions to determine whether seat belts and/or an airbag was involved.

Seat belts. Seat belts have prevented many thousands of injuries and have saved countless thousands of lives. Patients who otherwise would have been thrown out of a smashed car owe their lives to seat belts. However, if the

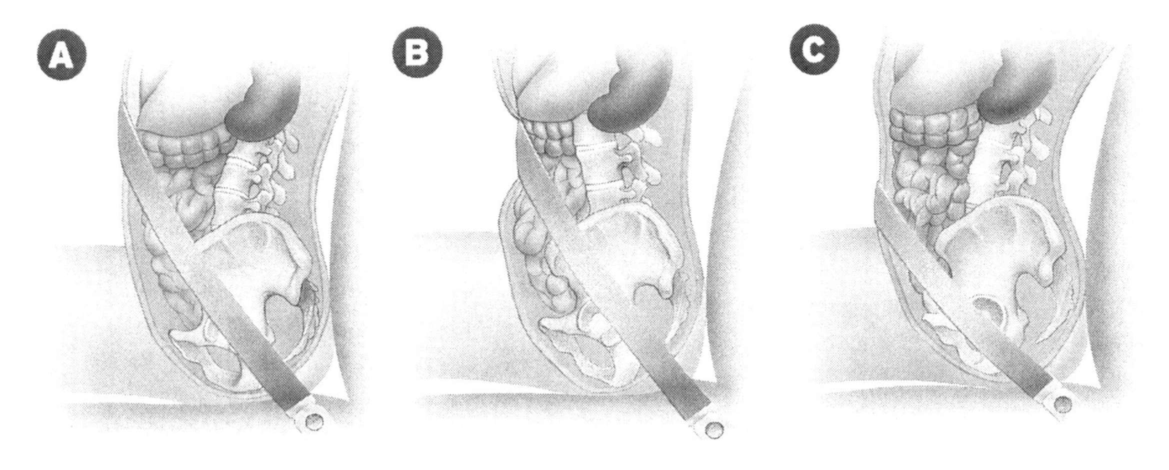

FIGURE 8-17 **A:** Injury may occur if the seat belt is placed too far above the iliac crest. **B:** A sudden stop could cause compression of the organs between the belt and the spine. **C:** The proper location of the seat belt is at the hip joints.

force of a crash is great enough, patients can have bruises under the seat belts and possible internal injuries, although these injuries are less severe than the injuries the patients would have sustained if they had not been wearing seat belts. Seat belts that are worn improperly across the abdomen rather than across the pelvic bones increase the potential for internal injuries (Figure 8-17). Lap seat belts must be worn so that they lie below the iliac crests, snugly up against the hip joints. If the seat belt is worn too high, sudden slowing or an abrupt stop might result in abdominal injuries. Occasionally, injuries of the lumbar spine can occur, even if the patient is wearing the seat belt properly.

Lap belts and shoulder belts are now commonly combined into a single unit. Some cars still have separate lap and shoulder belts. Used without a lap belt, shoulder belts can cause injuries of the chest, ribs, and liver.

Airbags. Airbags represent a great advance in automotive safety. Before airbags were common, individuals in head-on crashes would have significant facial injuries and bleeding—clear, visible signs that they had been injured. With airbags, patients occasionally have facial burns or respiratory problems from the chemical process that causes the airbag to expand, or they may have abrasions from the airbag itself. However, with airbags and seat belts, patients may or may not have visible injuries. Remember, while patients who have been involved in serious accidents may look fine, they may have internal injuries.

When an airbag deploys, a patient who is not wearing a seat belt can still go up and over, or down and under, the steering column. You should always look under a deployed air bag to see whether the steering wheel is bent or deformed in any way (Figure 8-18). Remove the patient from the car, using spinal precautions if indicated by patient complaint or mechanism of injury. If the wheel is bent or deformed in any way, you should suspect possible internal injuries. Internal injuries may also be possible if the steering wheel is not bent or deformed. The general health of the patient, the patient's age, and other factors can also impact the likelihood for internal injuries.

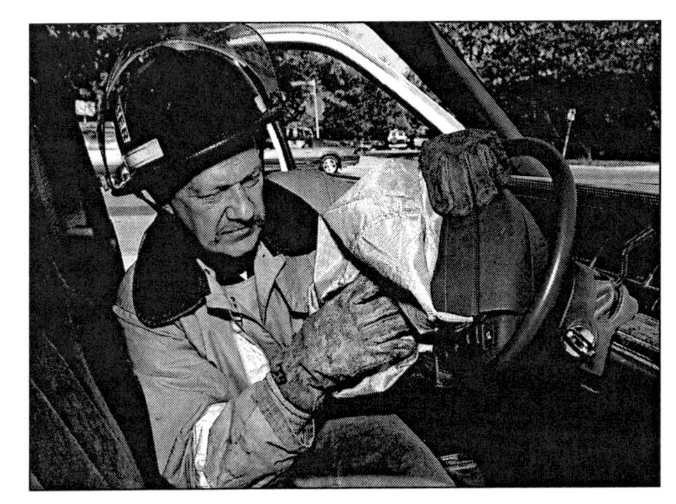

FIGURE 8-18 If an airbag has deployed, you should lift the airbag and check the steering wheel to see whether it is bent.

During your hand-off report at the hospital, make sure that you tell hospital personnel whether seat belts were worn—and if so, whether they were worn correctly (if you can tell)—and whether the airbag deployed.

Understanding the mechanism of injury helps you to estimate the severity of the patient's problem.

3

Trauma Patients With Significant Mechanism of Injury (MOI)

The rapid trauma assessment should be performed on any patient with significant mechanism of injury (MOI), to identify serious injuries that you were not concerned with during the initial assessment. The purpose of the rapid trauma assessment is to zero in on the patient's problems, as well as identify potentially life-threatening conditions, which will direct your physical exam. The rapid trauma assessment should be performed on responsive and unresponsive patients alike, who have suffered a significant MOI. Remember, you can use a responsive patient as a resource; you should ask him or her about symptoms throughout your assessment.

An integral part of this assessment is evaluation using the simple mnemonic "DCAP-BTLS." For each area of the body, you should quickly look for Deformities, Contusions, Abrasions, Punctures/Penetrations, Burns, Tenderness, Lacerations, and Swelling (DCAP-BTLS). Remember, you should interrupt your assessment to stabilize any immediately or potentially life-threatening conditions. Once these conditions have been stabilized, you may continue with your assessment.

Patient Assessment Process

Trauma Patient with a Significant Mechanism of Injury	Trauma Patient with No Significant Mechanism of Injury
Scene Size-Up	
Initial Assessment	
Focused History/Physical Exam*	
• Reconsider mechanism of injury	• Assess chief complaint
• Rapid trauma assessment	• Focused assessment of area of complaint
• Baseline vital signs	• Baseline vital signs
• SAMPLE history	• SAMPLE history
Detailed Physical Exam	
• Area by area exam*	
On-Going Assessment*	

* As appropriate

Rapid Trauma Assessment

1. **Check the patient's ABC** for any changes in status since the initial assessment.
2. **Continue spinal stabilization.**
3. **Re-Assess mental status.**
4. **Reconsider your transport decision,** if necessary.
5. **Consider a request for ALS backup.**
6. **Assess the head,** looking for DCAP-BTLS and crepitation.
7. **Assess the neck,** looking for DCAP-BTLS, jugular vein distention, and crepitation.
8. **Measure and apply** a cervical spinal immobilization collar.
9. **Assess the chest,** looking for DCAP-BTLS, paradoxical motion, and crepitation.. You should also assess for breath sounds in the apices, at the midclavicular line bilaterally, at the bases, and at the midaxillary line bilaterally.
10. **Assess the abdomen,** looking for DCAP-BTLS, rigidity (firm or soft), and distention.
11. **Assess the pelvis,** looking for DCAP-BTLS. If there is no pain, gently compress the pelvis downward or inward to determine tenderness or instability.
12. **Assess all four extremities,** looking for DCAP-BTLS. Also assess and compare bilaterally for distal pulses, sensation, and motor function.
13. **Roll the patient with spinal precautions,** and assess the posterior aspect of the body, looking for DCAP-BTLS. Position the long backboard and using spinal precautions, roll the patient supine onto the long backboard. While another trained prehospital care provider secures the patient to the long backboard, you can continue the focused history and physical exam.
14. **Assess baseline vital signs.**
15. **Assess the SAMPLE history.**

Recognizing a possible spinal injury is one of your principal responsibilities as a prehospital care provider. You should assume a spinal injury in any patient who has a mechanism of injury that reflects or suggests a significant history of trauma, is intoxicated and may have been traumatized, is unconscious, complains of neck/spine pain following a traumatic event, or cannot move or feel in any or all four extremities following a traumatic event. Immediately begin manual stabilization of the spine. Consider requesting ALS backup or transporting the patient with priority status. Also reevaluate the patient's mental status. Table 8-6 lists the conditions for which you should assess in addition to DCAP-BTLS during the rapid trauma assessment.

Head, Neck, and Cervical Spine

Look for abnormalities of the head, neck, and cervical spine. Gently feel the head and the back of the neck for deformity, tenderness, or crepitation, also checking as you feel for any bleeding. Crepitation is the crackling sound that is often heard when two ends of a broken bone rub together or when there are air bubbles under the skin. Ask a responsive patient if he or she feels any pain or tenderness. Next, check the neck for signs of trauma, swelling, or bleeding. Feel the skin of the neck for air under the skin, known as subcutaneous emphysema (crepitation), as well as any abnormal lumps or masses. It is particularly important to evaluate the neck before covering it with a cervical collar. Also look for pronounced or distended jugular veins. This can be normal in a patient who is lying down; however, their presence in the patient who is sitting up suggests some problem with blood returning to the heart. Report and record your findings carefully. Do not move on to the next step until you are sure that the airway is secure and you have initiated or continued spinal immobilization procedures.

Chest

Next, look at and feel over the chest area for injury or signs of trauma, including bruising, tenderness, or swelling. Watch the chest rise and fall with breathing. Normal breathing causes both sides of the chest to rise and fall together. Look for abnormal breathing signs, including retractions (when the skin pulls in around the ribs during inspiration) or paradoxical motion (when only one side rises on inspiration while another area of the chest falls).

Retractions indicate that the patient has some condition, usually medical, that is impairing the flow of air into and out of the lungs. Paradoxical motion is associated with a condition in which three or more ribs are each fractured in two or more places, causing a section of the chest wall to move independently from the rest of the chest. Palpate for grating of bones as the patient breathes. Crepitation is associated with rib fractures. Palpate the chest for subcutaneous emphysema (presence of air under the skin), especially in cases of severe blunt chest trauma. The sensation of crackling or popping, not unlike palpating the bubbles in bubble-pack packing material, is called subcutaneous emphysema; it indicates that air is leaking into the space under the skin. Usually, this means that the patient has a pneumothorax or has damaged the larynx.

TABLE 8-6 Using DCAP-BTLS in the Rapid Trauma Assessment

Part of the Body	Look for DCAP-BTLS and the Following:
Head	• Crepitation
Neck	• Jugular vein distention • Crepitation
Chest	• Paradoxical motion • Crepitation • Quality of breath sounds
Abdomen	• Rigidity • Distention
Pelvis	• Tenderness • Instability
Extremities	• Distal pulses • Sensation • Motor function
Back	

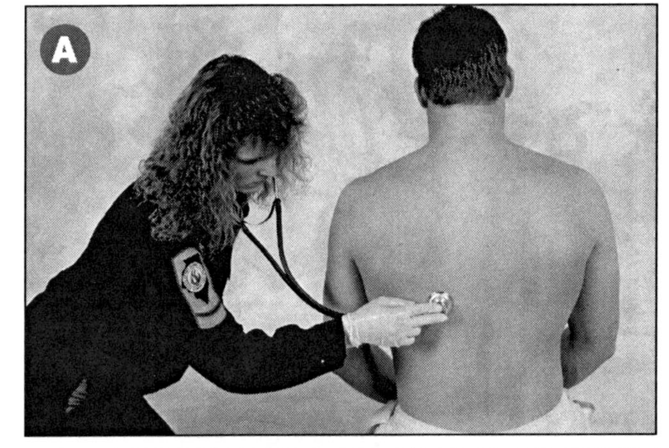

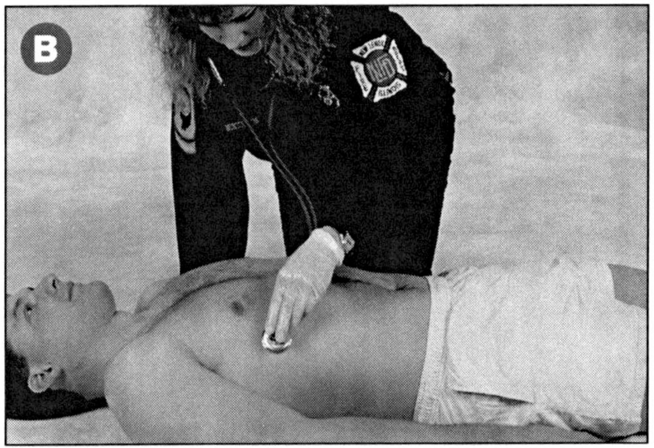

FIGURE 8-20 **A:** Listen to breath sounds from the patient's back if possible, over the apices, the bases, and the major airways. **B:** If the patient is immobilized or in a supine position, listen from the front.

3

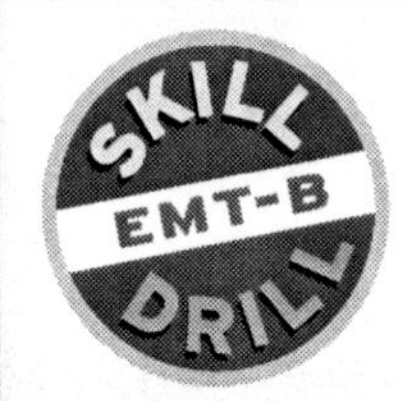

Performing a Rapid Trauma Assessment

Figure 8-19

1

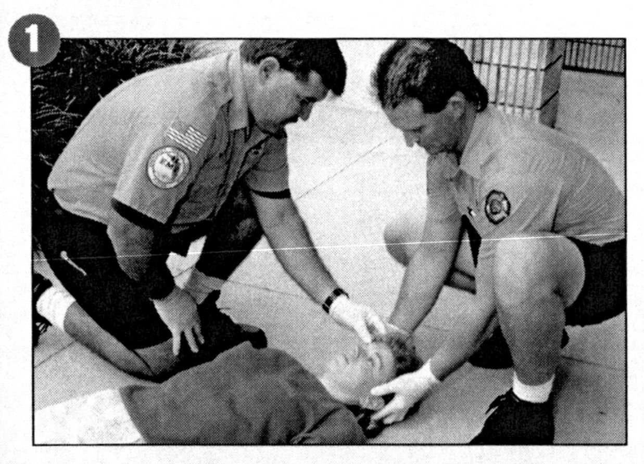

Assess the head for DCAP-BTLS and crepitation. Continue spinal stabilization

2

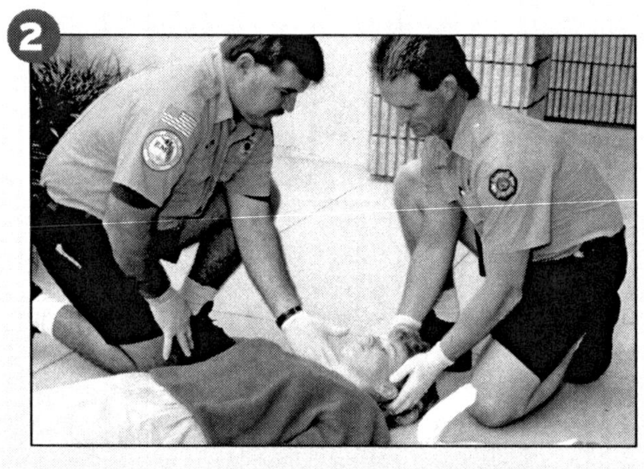

Assess the neck for DCAP-BTLS, jugular vein distention, and crepitation.

3

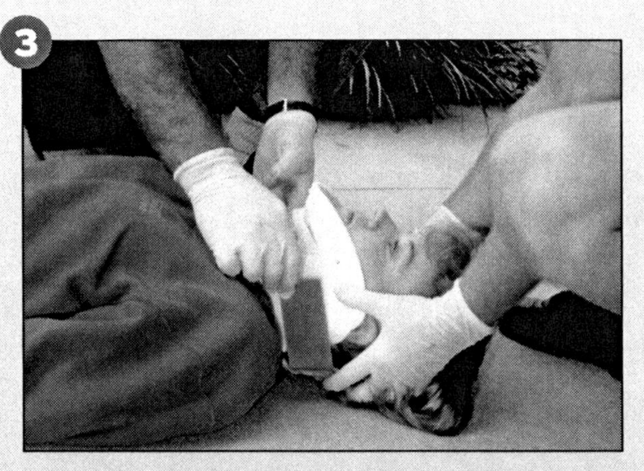

Measure and apply a cervical collar on the patient.

4

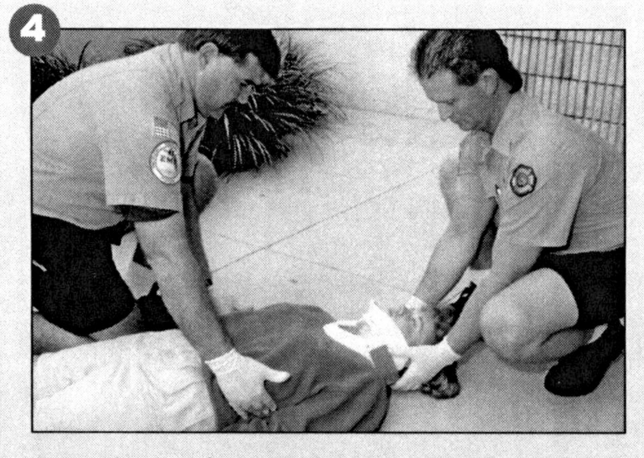

Assess the chest for DCAP-BTLS, paradoxical motion, and crepitation. Also assess for breath sounds.

5

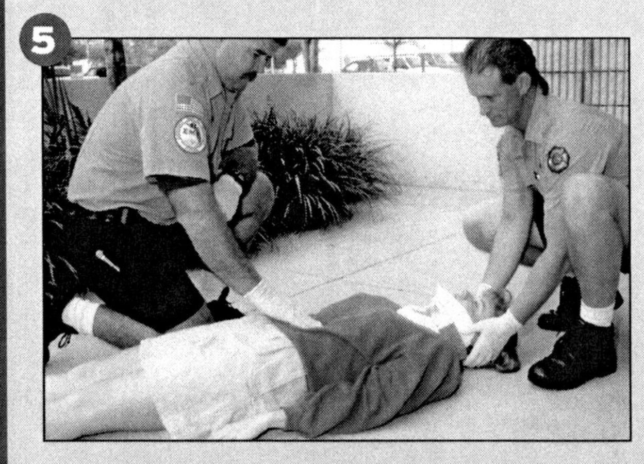

Assess the abdomen for DCAP-BTLS, rigidity, and distention.

6

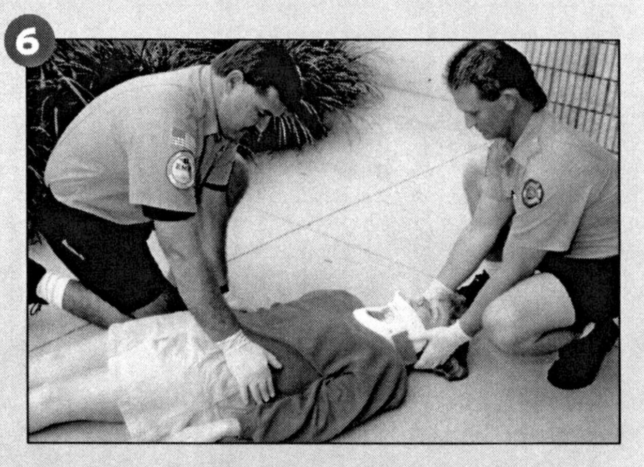

Assess the pelvis for DCAP-BTLS.

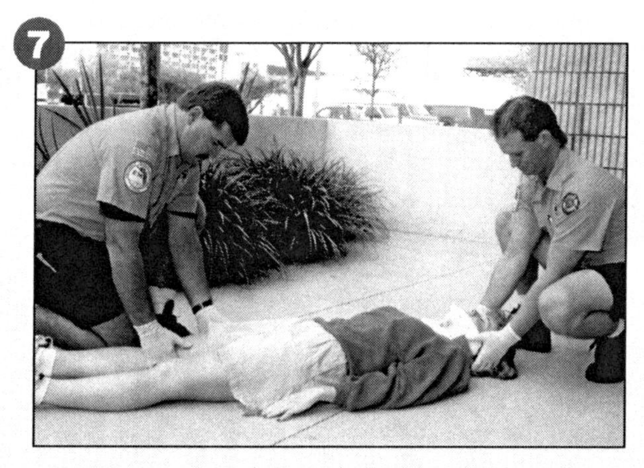

Assess all four extremities for DCAP-BTLS and distal pulse, motor and sensory.

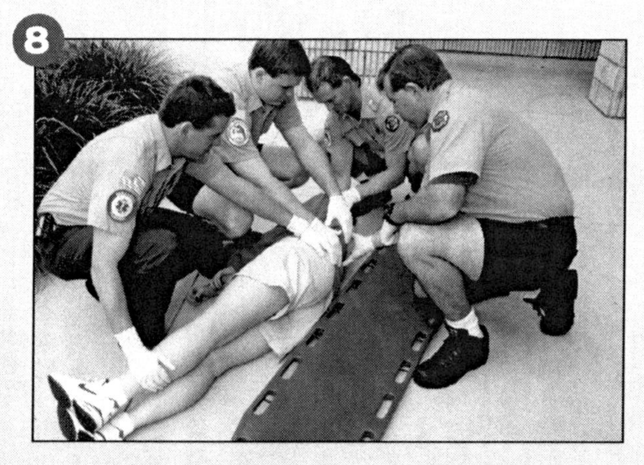

Roll the patient using spinal precautions, and assess the back for DCAP-BTLS.

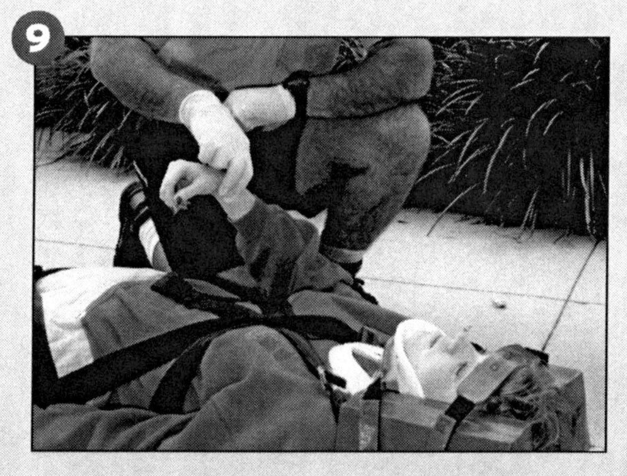

Assess baseline vitals and SAMPLE history.

If the patient reports difficulty breathing or has evidence of trauma to the chest, listen to **breath sounds**. This helps you to evaluate air movement in and out of the lungs. To listen, you need a stethoscope. Make sure that you place the earpieces facing forward in your ears. The anatomical position of the patient will determine the placement of the stethoscope to check for breath sounds (Figure 8-20).

Here's how and where to listen:

- First, remember that you can almost always hear breath sounds better from the patient's back. So if the patient's back is accessible, listen there. If you have immobilized the patient or if the patient is in a supine position and should not be moved, listen from the front.
- Listen over the upper lungs (apices), the lower lungs (bases), and over the major airways (midclavicular and midaxillary lines).
- Lift the clothing, or slide the stethoscope under the clothing. When you listen over clothing, you are hearing primarily the sound of the stethoscope sliding over the fabric, because the breath sounds are muted by the clothing.
- Place the diaphragm of the stethoscope firmly to best hear the breath sounds.

What are you listening for? Your goal is to hear and document the presence or absence of breath sounds in the three regions described. If you believe that the breathing is abnormal, recheck the initial assessment for adequate breathing, and ensure that the patient is receiving oxygen and, if appropriate, assisted ventilation.

Abdomen

Look at the abdomen for any obvious injuries, bruising, and bleeding. Be sure to feel over both the front and the sides of the abdomen, evaluating for tenderness and any bleeding. As you feel all around the abdomen, use the terms "firm," "soft," "tender," or "distended" (swollen) to report your findings. If the patient is awake and alert, ask about pain as you perform the exam. Do not palpate obvious soft-tissue injuries, and be careful not to palpate too hard.

Pelvis

Look for any signs of obvious injury, bleeding, or deformity. If the patient reports no pain, gently press inward and downward on the pelvic bones. Do not rock the pelvis, since this motion may move an unstable spine. If you feel any movement or crepitation, or the patient reports pain or tenderness, it may indicate severe injury. Injuries to the pelvis and surrounding abdomen may bleed profusely, so continue to monitor the patient's skin color, temperature, and condition, and be sure that you are giving supplemental oxygen.

Extremities

Using the mnemonic DCAP-BTLS, inspect and palpate each extremity for deformities, contusions, abrasions, penetrations/punctures, burns, tenderness, lacerations, and swelling. Ask the patient about any pain. As you evaluate the extremities, check for distal circulation, sensation, and movement:

- **Circulation:** Evaluate the skin color in the hands or feet. Is it normal? How does it compare with the skin color of the other extremities? Pale or cyanotic skin may indicate poor circulation in the extremity. Check the distal pulses on the foot (dorsalis pedis or posterior tibial) and wrist (radial).
- **Sensation:** Evaluate normal feeling in the extremity by asking the patient to close his or her eyes. Gently squeeze or pinch a finger or toe, and ask the patient to identify what you are doing. The inability to feel sensation in the extremity may indicate a local nerve injury. Inability to feel in several extremities may be a sign of spinal cord injury. Recheck to be sure that you have begun and/or are maintaining spinal immobilization.
- **Movement:** Ask the patient to wiggle his or her fingers or toes. An inability to move a single extremity can be the result of a bone, muscle, or nerve injury. Inability to move several extremities may be a sign of a brain abnormality or spinal cord injury. Recheck to be sure that you have initiated spinal immobilization.

3

Back

Palpate the back for DCAP-BTLS. If you are placing the patient on a backboard, it is particularly important that you check the back before you log roll the patient onto the backboard. Ensure that you keep the spine in line at all times as you log roll the patient onto his or her side. Carefully palpate the spine from the neck to the pelvis for tenderness or deformity, and visualize for obvious injuries, including bruising.

Baseline Vital Signs and SAMPLE History

After you have completed the rapid trauma assessment, it is time to obtain baseline vital signs and a SAMPLE history.

The baseline vital signs provide useful information about the overall functions of the patient's heart and lungs. They may be an important part of the focused history and physical examination if your patient appears to have problems related to blood loss, circulation, or breathing. In other cases, you may simply document the vital signs as baseline information. If the patient's condition is stable, you should reassess the vital signs every 15 minutes until you reach the emergency department. If the patient is categorized as a high priority patient, you should reassess at a minimum of every 5 minutes, or as often as the situation permits, looking for trends in the patient's condition. Tables 8-7 through 8-12 provide more information on baseline vital signs.

TABLE 8-7 Determining the Quality of Breathing

Normal	• Breathing is neither shallow nor deep. • Average chest wall motion • No use of accessory muscles
Shallow	• Slight chest or abdominal wall motion
Labored	• Increased breathing effort • Grunting, stridor • Use of accessory muscles • Gasping for air • Nasal flaring, supraclavicular and intercostal retractions (in infants and children)
Noisy	• Increase in sound of breathing, including snoring, wheezing, gurgling, and crowing

TABLE 8-8 Normal Respiration Rates

Adults	12 to 20 breaths/min
Children	15 to 30 breaths/min
Infants	25 to 50 breaths/min

TABLE 8-9 Average Pulse Rates

Adults	60 to 100 beats/min
Children	80 to 100 beats/min
Toddlers	100 to 120 beats/min

TABLE 8-10 Assessing the Skin

Color	Possible Cause
Pink	• Normal color
Ashen/White Face and/or Skin on Extremities	• Hypovolemia (blood loss)
Gray-Blue (cyanotic)	• Insufficient air exchange • Low blood oxygen levels
Flushed	• High blood pressure • Carbon monoxide poisoning • Significant fever • Heatstroke (life-threatening heat related emergency) • Sunburn • Mild thermal burns
Jaundice	• Liver disease or dysfunction
Temperature/Moisture	**Possible Cause**
Warm	• Normal condition
Hot	• Significant fever • Sunburn • Hyperthermia
Cool	• Early shock • Heavy exercise/sweating • Heat exhaustion
Cold	• Profound shock • Hypothermia • Frostbite
Dry	• Normal condition
Clammy, Damp, or Moist	• Early shock
Wet	• Profound shock

TABLE 8-11 Systolic Blood Pressure Readings

Expected Readings		Critically Low Readings	
Adult Men	Add 100 to the patient's age, up to 150 mm Hg	**Male Adults/ Adolescents**	90 mm Hg or less
Adult Women	Add 90 to the patient's age, up to 150 mm Hg	**Female Adults/ Adolescents**	80 mm Hg or less
Children	Add 80 to 2 times the patient's age in years	**Children**	70 mm Hg or less

TABLE 8-12 Pupillary Reactions

Appearance	Possible Cause
Round/equal size	Normal condition
Fixed with no reaction to light	Depressed brain function
Fully dilated and fixed (blown pupil)	Intracranial bleeding
Dilate with bright light, constricted with low light	Depressed brain function
Constricted	Opiates in system
Sluggish reaction	Depressed brain function
Unequal in size	Depressed brain function Medication placed in eye Injury or condition of the eye
Unequal in size when bright light is introduced	Depressed brain function or removed from one eye

Do not be falsely reassured by apparently normal vital signs. The body has amazing abilities to compensate for severe injury or illness, especially in children and young adults. Even patients with severe medical or traumatic conditions may initially present with fairly normal vital signs. However, the body eventually loses its ability to compensate, and the vital signs may suddenly deteriorate rapidly, especially in children. In fact, this tendency for the vital signs to fall rapidly as the patient decompensates is the reason that it is important to frequently recheck and record the vital signs.

For many prehospital care providers, taking the patient history seems to be a bewildering series of questions that seem to bear little or no relationship to the patient's need for help. This becomes worse with patients who have had many medical problems; taking their history is time consuming and often yields little or no information that is useful to you. However, this does not need to be the case. Remember that the mnemonic SAMPLE includes the following elements:

Signs and Symptoms of the episode

Allergies, particularly to medications

Medications, including prescription, over-the-counter, and recreational (illicit) drugs

Pertinent past medical history, particularly involving similar episodes in the past

Last oral intake, including medications, as well as food and/or drinks. This is particularly important if the patient may need surgery

Events leading up to the episode, which may include precipitating factors

Trauma Patients With No Significant Mechanism of Injury

You will not need to perform a rapid trauma assessment on all of your patients who are victims of trauma. During the first step of the focused history and physical exam: trauma, you will re-consider the mechanism of injury (MOI) to determine if the patient requires a rapid trauma assessment or the focused trauma assessment. If you determine that the patient is *not* a high priority patient and did *not* suffer a significant MOI, then you should focus your attention on anything associated with the patient's specific injury site or chief complaint and perform the focused assessment. The focused assessment is performed in lieu of the rapid trauma assessment, to further examine a minor or isolated injury on a victim of trauma with no significant mechanism of injury.

Assess the Chief Complaint

Start by examining problems associated with the chief complaint: the patient's description of "what is wrong." For example, if the patient reports ankle pain, you should inspect and palpate the ankle for DCAP-BTLS, unstable movement, and distal pulse, motor, and sensory. Note, though, that nontraumatic complaints may be a little less obvious. Here are some things to assess with some common chief complaints:

- **Chest pain:** Evaluate the skin color, temperature and condition, pulse, and blood pressure. Inspect and palpate the chest for DCAP-BTLS, crepitation, and listen to breath sounds.

- **Shortness of breath:** Evaluate the skin color, temperature and condition, pulse, blood pressure, and rate and depth of respirations. Look for signs of airway obstruction, as well as trauma to the neck and chest. Listen carefully to the breath sounds.
- **Abdominal pain:** Evaluate the skin color, temperature and condition, pulse and blood pressure. Inspect and palpate for DCAP-BTLS, and palpate the abdomen to identify any particularly tender spots.
- **Any pain associated with bones or joints:** Evaluate the skin color, temperature and condition, and distal pulse, motor and sensory. Inspect and palpate the area for DCAP-BTLS.
- **Dizziness:** Evaluate the skin color, temperature and condition, pulse, blood pressure, and rate and quality of respirations. Monitor the level of consciousness and orientation carefully. Assess the head for DCAP-BTLS.

Once you have examined chief complaints, you can come back to any minor problems you found previously. Be sure to ask the patient questions about the abnormality while you are evaluating it. In some cases, deformities or abnormalities may be long-term and unrelated to the patient's present condition. For example, a patient who has had a stroke may have a weakness on one side for months following the stroke; it is not a new problem, and it is not likely to be related to the patient's current call for EMS.

Perform a Focused Assessment

As we have noted before, plan ahead for BSI; if bleeding is possible (and it is for most victims of trauma), be sure your gloves are on before you begin the focused examination. Next, inspect and palpate the specific area of injury or complaint for DCAP-BTLS and any other signs of injury.

Obtain Baseline Vital Signs and SAMPLE History

As you know, baseline vital signs provide useful information about the overall functions of the patient's heart and lungs. Remember, if the patient's condition is stable, you should reassess the vital signs every 15 minutes until you reach the emergency department. If the patient is unstable, you should reassess at a minimum of every 5 minutes, or as often as the situation permits. Also obtain a SAMPLE history if possible.

Documentation

Baseline findings during this examination document how the patient looked during your assessment. Your written report should include documentation of the following:

- Findings and interventions from the initial assessment
- Findings and interventions from the rapid trauma assessment or focused trauma assessment, including pertinent negatives
- Baseline vital signs (respirations, pulse, blood pressure, skin CTC, and pupils)
- SAMPLE history

Other Considerations

Remember, for many patients, you will need to assess the entire body because of the potential severity of their condition. The following patients require a complete rapid trauma assessment, coupled with short scene time and rapid transport to the hospital:

- Any patients who experienced a significant mechanism of injury
- Any patients who are unresponsive or disoriented, since they cannot contribute to the focused history and physical exam
- Any patients who are extremely intoxicated from drugs or alcohol and cannot reliably contribute to the focused history and physical exam

Any patients with a complaint that cannot be identified or clearly understood by using a focused physical exam should receive a more complete exam.

Focused History and Physical Exam: Medical Patients

This component of patient assessment is performed after making the determination that there is no mechanism of injury; there is no trauma. During the focused history and physical exam: medical, the mnemonic **OPQRST** and **SAMPLE** will be used to gather information about the chief complaint and history of present illness. Baseline vital signs and a focused physical exam *or* a rapid medical assessment will also be performed. The order in which you perform the steps of the focused history and physical exam: medical patient varies depending on whether the patient is responsive or unresponsive.

Before you begin the focused history and physical exam: medical you would have received the dispatch information and information from both the scene size-up and initial assessment. These have provided you with valuable information about the scene, allowing you to anticipate what you will find and prepare for hazards. If your patient had problems with ABC, you have stabilized any life-threatening conditions during the initial assessment, and have begun transport procedures. How do you proceed now? Your patient may have, almost literally, one or more of a million different problems. How do you identify, prioritize, and treat this variety of potential problems? Early in the assessment process, you need to begin evaluating the patient's problem. In most cases, the patient is alert and able to discuss the problem with you. However, in some cases, the patient may be confused, intoxicated, unable to speak your language, or unconscious. In such a situation, you should immediately proceed to the rapid medical assessment.

When the patient can tell you about his or her problem, the response to general questions such as "What's wrong?" or "What happened?" is called the chief complaint. This is what drives your assessment of the history of the present illness. The chief complaint is typically the problem that is bothering the patient the most, and the question "What's wrong?" or "What happened?" is one of the most critical questions you can ask.

Be careful not to jump to conclusions regarding the chief complaint because of what you have seen or heard about the patient. There are cases in which the chief complaint will not be obvious; it may even be different from what the dispatcher reported. When this occurs, stay flexible. Treat the patient's problem rather than simply reacting to the dispatch report. Nevertheless, the chief complaint represents what is bothering the patient and will help you to focus your history and physical exam.

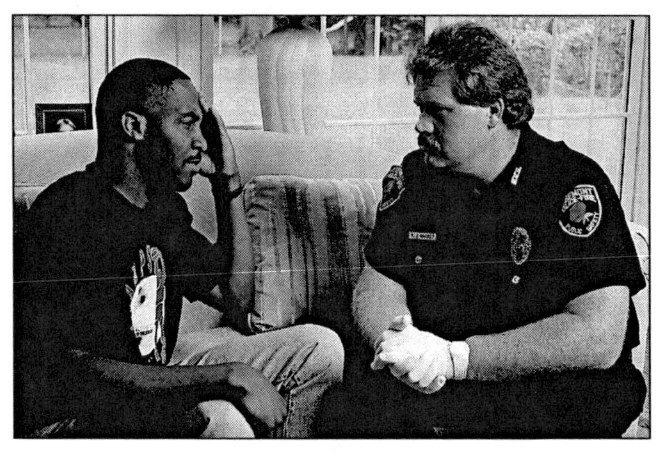

FIGURE 8-21 The patient's initial response to the question "What's wrong?" is the chief complaint.

Assessing the Responsive Patient

The key to truly understanding a patient's chief complaint is to ask open-ended questions such as "What seems to be the problem?" or "What's wrong?" and then listening (Figure 8-21). This is where good communication skills really pay off. If possible, take the time to sit down and help the patient to get comfortable. Now is the time to listen, as you develop an increased understanding of the patient's real problems. If the patient cannot tell you what is wrong, perhaps because of a language barrier, altered mental status, or severe respiratory difficulty, you may learn the chief complaint from a family member or bystander or from your observations of the scene and patient actions. However, remember that information directly from the patient is far more valuable. You should try, whenever possible, to speak directly to the patient.

As you listen to the patient, you might want to make some brief notes to aid your memory and assist with documentation after the call. You should attempt to record the chief complaint in a few of the patient's own words. Be sure to note if your information comes from someone other than the patient.

PATIENT ASSESSMENT FLOWCHART

Focused History and Physical Exam: Medical Patients

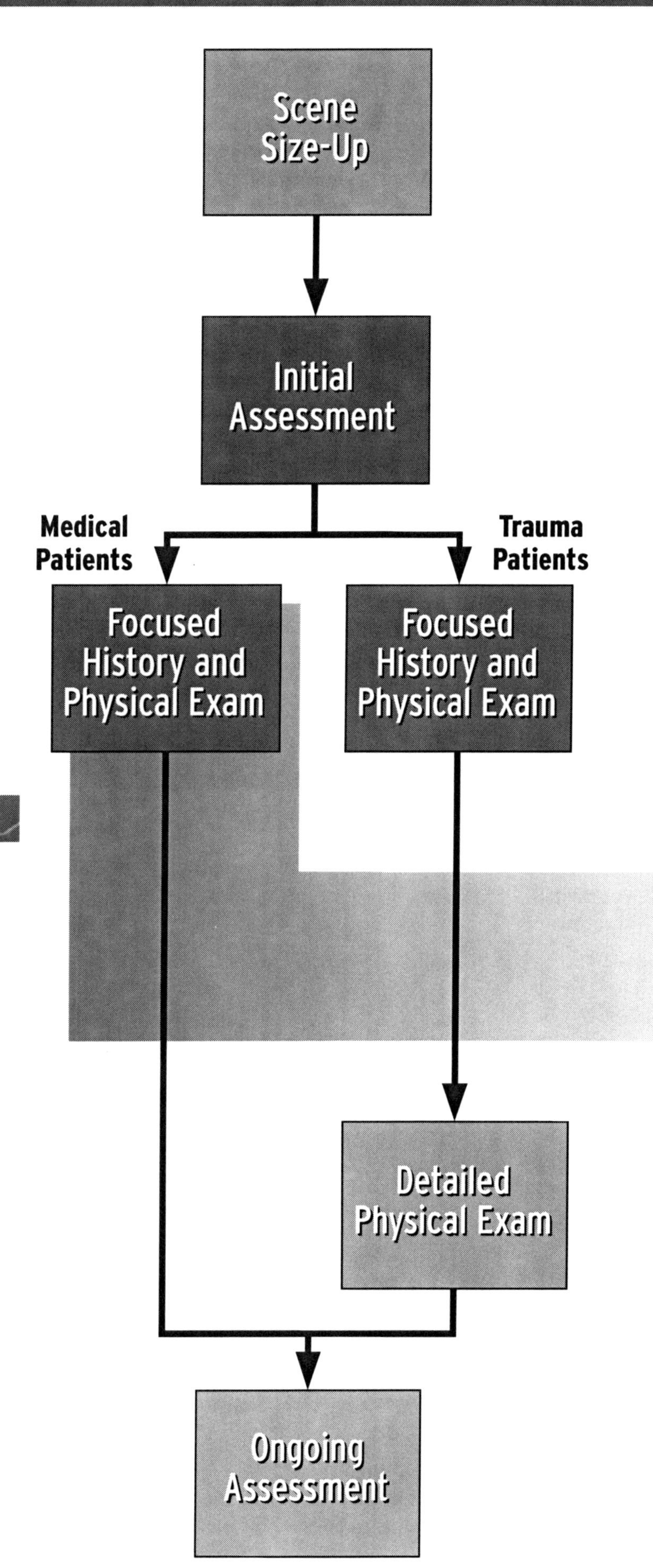

ient Assessment Process

ɪdical Patient ɔ Is Responsive	Medical Patient Who Is Not Responsive
Scene Size-Up	
Initial Assessment	
Focused History/Physical Exam*	
ɜsess chief ·mplaint -P-Q-R-S-T ɅMPLE ːom family or ʼstanders) ɔcused physical ːam ɪseline vital signs	• Rapid medical assessment • Baseline vital signs • OPQRST and SAMPLE history
Detailed Physical Exam	
ot a candidate	• As needed (do not delay transport
On-Going Assessment*	
ɪile enroute to the hospital	

4

OPQRST

As you learn about the chief complaint, you should broaden your knowledge to include the circumstances surrounding the complaint. You can remember the six most important circumstances by using the letters OPQRST, which stand for **O**nset, **P**rovocation, **Q**uality, **R**adiation, **S**everity, and **T**ime. Table 8-13 lists the components of the focused history and physical exam for the medical patient.

Onset. The onset refers to what the patient was doing when the problem first began. You should ask the patient what he/she was doing when the problem first started. Was the patient at rest when the signs and symptoms started? Sitting in a chair watching TV? Awoken in the middle of the night by the problem?, etc. The answer to these questions often helps you to appreciate the potential cause. For instance, shortness of breath that started when the patient climbed a set of stairs may be respiratory or cardiac in origin. However, shortness of breath that started after the patient was struck in the chest by a baseball might be the result of fractured ribs or internal injury. These questions are often the clues to hidden medical problems in traumatic incidents, such as the patient who reports that she fell down the stairs because she felt "real dizzy." "O" for onset cues your memory to ask, "What were you doing when this started?"

Provocation. Learning about provoking factors can be extremely helpful in determining the cause and seriousness of the presenting problem. Provoking factors include anything that seems to bring on the problem or that seems to makes the problem worse. After determining what the patient was doing when the problem started, what he or she thinks caused the problem, you should then ask the patient what, if anything, makes the problem better or worse. Does the patient feel some relief of symptoms when resting? Does the patient feel some relief of symptoms after taking prescribed medication? Are the symptoms worse when the patient takes a deep breath?, etc. "P" for provocation cues your memory to ask, "Is there anything that makes you feel better or worse?"

TABLE 8-13 Components of the Focused History and Physical Exam: Medical Patient

Responsive Patient	Unresponsive Patient
• Use OPQRST to gather a history of the patient's problem: Onset Provocation Quality Radiation Severity Time • Obtain present and past medical history (SAMPLE): Signs and symptoms Allergies Medications Past history Last oral intake Events leading up to the episode • Perform a focused exam: Identify potentially life-threatening conditions Examine areas related to the chief complaint Noticeable abnormalities • Obtain baseline vital signs: Reassess every 15 minutes in a stable patient Reassess every 5 minutes in an unstable patient	• Perform a rapid medical assessment: Head Neck Chest Abdomen Pelvis Extremities Back • Obtain baseline vital signs. • Provide emergency medical care and transport: Ask the family about the chief complaint, the history of present illness, and SAMPLE while enroute to the hospital. • Document your findings: Initial assessment Were there any life threats? Focused history and physical exam Note pertinent positive and negative signs and symptoms

Quality of pain. The patient's description of pain may be very useful to hospital staff who are trying to determine the cause of the problem. For instance, patients who are having a heart attack frequently describe their chest pain as "squeezing" or "pressure," although they may also say things like, "I feel funny," for lack of having a better description or, "I just don't feel well." To learn about the quality of pain, ask the patient to describe the pain or explain what the pain feels like to them.

Patients will often initially say, "I don't know," or "It's hard to describe." Once again, the key is for you to be patient. If you wait, most patients will ultimately describe the quality of their pain. Carefully document the patient's own words; these may be very significant to other providers who become involved in the patient's care. If the patient still cannot describe the pain, or if the patient cannot speak, you might consider offering several descriptions of pain and letting the patient choose. For instance, you might ask, "Which of these words best describes your pain: Sharp or dull? Burning, stabbing, crushing, or throbbing?" "Q" for quality cues your memory to ask, "What does the pain feel like?"

Radiation. Patients can often provide clues about the cause of their problems by describing the region or location of any pain or discomfort (Figure 8-22). Radiation refers to any additional area where the pain or discomfort may also be present. The presence of radiating pain will not alter your treatment very much; however, physicians and nurses caring for the patient in the hospital may be very interested in hearing about areas of radiation. For example, a patient who is having a heart attack may report chest pain that radiates to the left arm and jaw. Document carefully what you learn.

Some patients have limited vocabulary when it comes to their bodies; it may be best to let them simply point to their pain, rather than describe it. Ask patients to point to the area of pain, describe the area of pain, or describe pain anywhere else associated with the problem.

You can learn a great deal about the patient's problem through these questions. For instance, a patient who points to a single place for his or her pain has what is known as focal pain. Many problems, such as fractures or inflammations, are classically focal. However, some patients cannot point to a single location. Instead, they often move their finger around in a circle as they are asked to point to their pain. These patients are experiencing diffuse pain. A number of conditions, including heart attack and internal bleeding, are typically diffuse.

Be careful how you ask about radiation of pain. Most patients will not understand if you ask, "Does your pain radiate anywhere else?" And asking, "Does your pain go (or travel) anywhere else?" might confuse the patient. "R" for radiation cues your memory to ask, "Where do you feel the pain? Can you point to it with one finger? Do you have pain anywhere else?"

Severity. Severity refers to the patient's perception of "how bad" the current incident is in comparison to

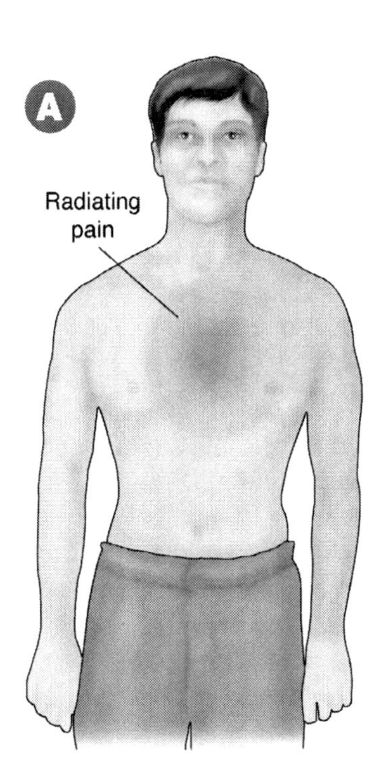

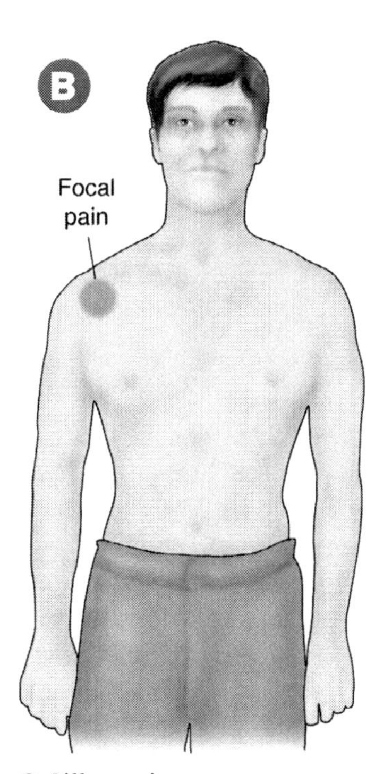

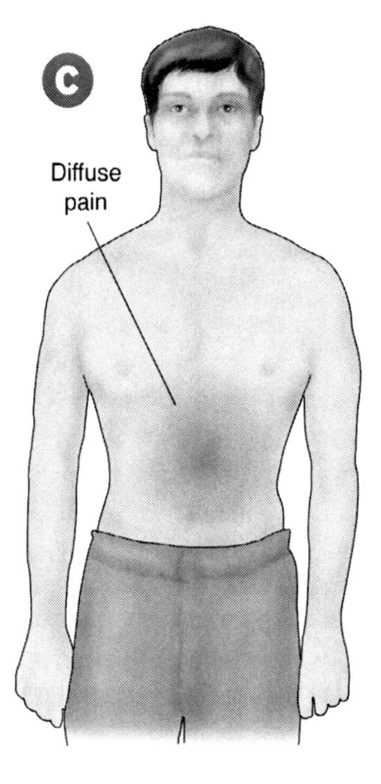

FIGURE 8-22 **A:** Radiating pain. **B:** Focal pain. **C:** Diffuse pain.

4

others. In some cases, particularly when the patient has experienced the problem before, his or her perception provides extremely useful information. For example, a patient with asthma may be very helpful by comparing this episode with other previous asthma attacks. However, if the problem has never occurred, the patient's perception may not be very useful except as a guide to whether it is getting worse or better during transport. To assess severity, you may ask the following questions:

- "How bad is this episode in comparison to previous ones?" (if the problem is chronic or recurring).
- "What happened the last time you had an episode this bad?" (if the problem is chronic or recurring).
- "How would you rate this problem in numbers, if 1 is normal and 10 is the worst pain or discomfort you can imagine?"

For patients with chronic problems, obtaining the answer to the question "What happened the last time you had an episode this bad?" is invaluable. In most cases, patients have been found to be very accurate in their self-assessments of severity. For instance, a patient with asthma might tell you that the last time he had an attack this bad, he was in the hospital for two weeks, with one week in the intensive care unit. The patient's comments tell you that this episode is extremely serious and that you should complete your assessment and provide immediate transport. At the other extreme, the patient might tell you that he was kept in the emergency department for about an hour and then discharged. Obviously, these two episodes are very different in urgency, and you can adjust your plans for treatment and transport accordingly.

Another way to evaluate changes in the patient's condition during your treatment and transport is to use a numerical score system. For example, a patient with an apparent broken leg might initially tell you that the pain is an 8 on a scale of 1 to 10. After you splint the leg and begin transport, you should recheck the patient's perception. If the pain is now a 9, you might consider changing the position of the leg or using an ice pack. However, if the pain level is now reportedly a 5, you know that the treatment is effective, at least for now. Remember, patients perceive pain in different ways, so it is inappropriate to compare one patient's numerical score with another patient's score. "S" for severity cues your memory to ask, "How bad is the pain? How would you rate the pain on a scale of 1-10, with 10 being the worst pain you have ever felt?"

Time. The final set of questions asked, using the mnemonic OPQRST, provides information about how long the patient has had these complaints. Has the problem been constant or intermittent. Did the problem occur suddenly or has this been occurring for several hours to days?

If the patient states that the problem is intermittent, ask about what seemed to make it better or worse. You might also ask what the patient has done independently to make it feel better. Did the patient's interventions help?

The answers to these questions will further help you and other health professionals involved with the patient's care to understand the nature of the problem. Some conditions, such as those involving abdominal organs, have classically intermittent pain. Other problems, such as fractures, typically have constant pain. Learning what the patient tried doing to make the problem better might also be very insightful. For instance, some patients smear butter on burns. The greasy wetness of the butter may make the burn look worse than it really is, and the salt in the butter usually intensifies the pain. Also, some patients may take too much medication to try to relieve pain. This may signal another problem: a potential overdose.

If the patient reports that the problem started a long time ago (days or weeks), you should also ask, "What made you finally call for help?" In most cases, the patient will note a sudden worsening of the problem or an additional problem that compounded the first one. For example, the patient complaining of shortness of breath for the past 3 days may have called because of a sudden onset of chest pain. You often will not learn about something like this unless you ask.

For patients with traumatic problems, there may be a delay between when they were hurt and when they called. Again, ask them why they had not called for help sooner, and what finally caused them to call. The information that they give you may be valuable to you or the hospital staff. "T" for time cues your memory to ask, "How long have you had this complaint?"

Other Questions to Consider

After you have evaluated the chief complaint using OPQRST, you need to ask three more questions pertaining to the chief complaint. Often, because of the intensity of a particular complaint, patients may be unaware or fail to mention other problems. These omissions are usually not serious. However, if the patient fails to mention a potentially life-threatening problem, you could miss an important symptom. For this reason, you should conclude your evaluation of the chief complaint by asking the following three questions:

additional follow-up questions

If you have time, you might find it helpful to ask this series of additional questions.

- **"Has this ever happened before?"** This question is very useful in that many patient will be experiencing flare-ups of previously existing problems. If the answer to this question is "yes," you should follow up with additional questions to understand the nature of this episode.
- **"Did you see the doctor or go to the hospital when it happened before?** If so, did the doctor tell you the name of what was wrong? What was it?" The goal here is to learn the patient's diagnosis.
- **"Do you take any medications for this problem?"** If the answer is "yes," then you might want to ask additional questions to determine what prescription and/or over-the-counter medications the patient is taking for the condition. Also ask to see the bottles or containers so that you can take them with you to the emergency department.

You need to ask questions about alcohol and illicit drug use, no matter where you work in EMS. Alcoholism and drug addiction affect all populations, from the wealthiest executive to the poorest of the poor. All races and ethnic groups are affected, too. How you ask these questions will vary from place to place, depending on the patient population that you serve. It is essential that you know the local culture and the terms that are used for alcohol and drug use. Learn how to ask these questions by watching and learning the approach that is used by other EMTs, paramedics, nurses, and doctors in your community. You are trying to obtain important information by asking the following questions:

- **"Are you a heavy alcohol user?** If so, when was your last drink?" Intoxication affects all other aspects of the history and physical exam. The symptoms of alcohol withdrawal are also important to note in conjunction with the patient's presentation.
- **"Do you use illicit drugs?** Which ones?" If the answer is yes, when was the patient's last "high"? Is he or she high now? These findings affect the remainder of the exam. Symptoms of drug withdrawal may complicate the patient's clinical picture by presenting different symptoms. Remember, your role is not law enforcement. You must gain the patient's trust so that you can provide the necessary emergency medical care. Assure the patient that your communication is confidential but that you need this information so that you can fully understanding his or her medical problem.
- **"Do you have any other problems I should know about?"** This question is handy to ask whether the patient has ever had this problem or not. It gives the patient an opportunity to tell you something about apparently unrelated previous medical problems. In most cases, the answer will serve as useful background information. Occasionally, it will provide you and the hospital with essential information.

4

1. **"Are you sure that you did not pass out?"** Changes in mental status are serious signs associated with brain injury or trauma. Try to make sure the patient never lost consciousness before, during, or after the injury or illness.
2. **"Are you sure that you are not having any difficulty breathing?"** Most patients with shortness of breath will complain about it early and often. However, patients are occasionally unaware of, or fail to mention, their difficulty in breathing, especially if they are in extreme pain. Respiratory problems may have severe consequences, so be sure that your patient is not having any difficulty breathing.
3. **"Are you certain that you are not experiencing any chest pain or discomfort?"** As with respiratory problems, most patients with chest pain will report it to you. However, some patients either do not complain about pain or are not aware of their chest discomfort. Yet chest pain may be a symptom of a serious cardiac problem, so it is essential that you do not miss it.

The SAMPLE History

Once you have obtained a clearer picture of the patient's chief complaint and have explored it using the OPQRST questions, you should obtain a SAMPLE history. Recall

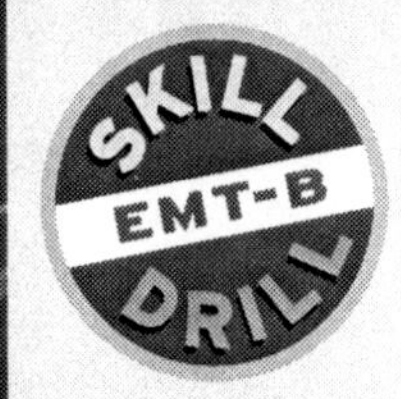

Performing a Focused Exam: Medical Patient

Figure 8-23

1

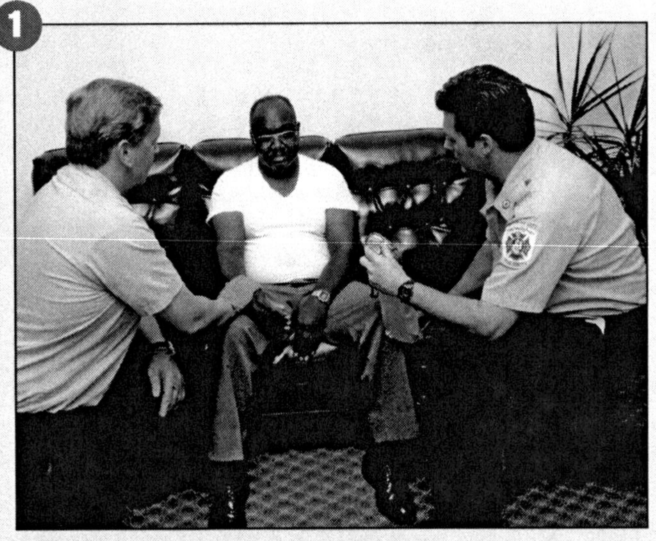

Assess for any potentially life-threatening conditions, followed by problems associated with the chief complaint.

2

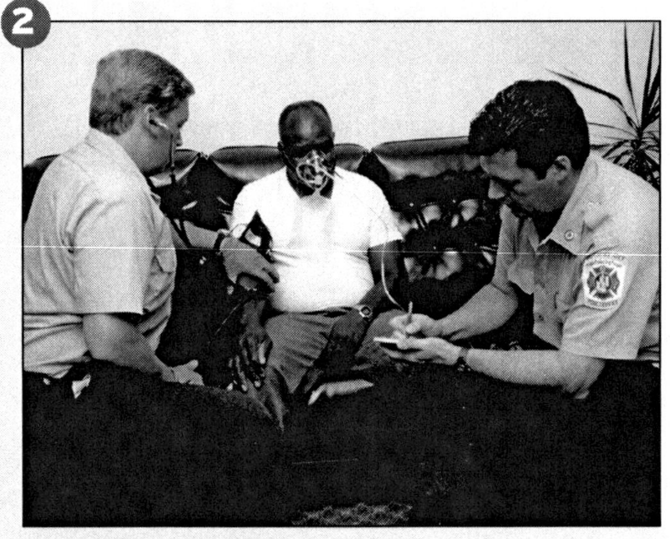

Obtain baseline vital signs, and document your findings.

3

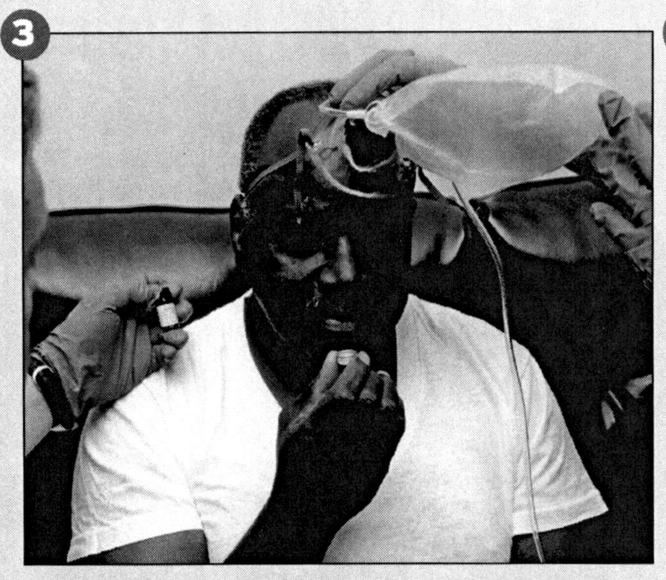

Provide emergency care for life-threatening or serious conditions as well as treatment for the chief complaint.

4

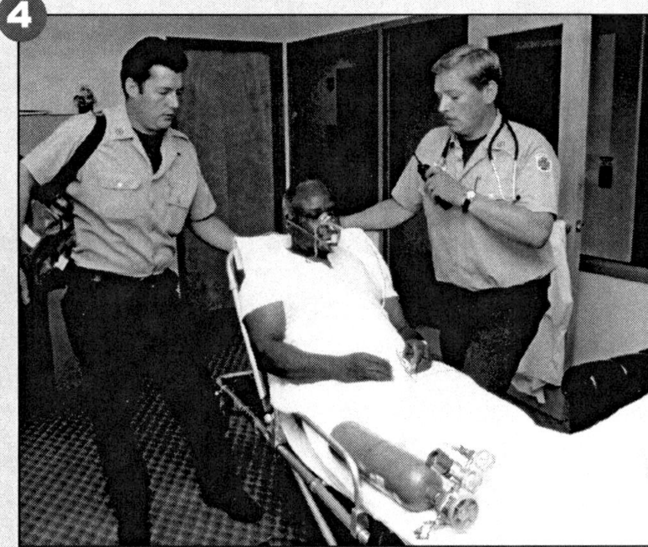

Transport the patient.

that the purpose of this history is to gather information about the patient's present and past medical experiences. The elements of the SAMPLE history are repeated below for your review.

- **S**igns and **S**ymptoms of the episode
- **A**llergies, particularly to medications
- **M**edications, including prescription, over-the-counter, and recreational (illicit) drugs
- **P**ertinent past history, especially involving similar episodes in the past
- **L**ast oral intake, including food and/or drinks. This is particularly important if the patient may need surgery. Also determine if the patient has taken prescribed medication as directed.
- **E**vents leading up to the episode, which may include precipitating factors (this question may be redundant with "O" onset).

You should also ask whether the patient has any other problems that you should know about. This question is useful in that it gives the patient an opportunity to tell you something about seemingly unrelated previous medical problems. In most cases, this will serve as useful background information. Occasionally, it will provide you and hospital staff with essential information, such as when you discovered that the patient who fell for no apparent reason has a history of diabetes. This information suggests the possibility that the fall was caused by a complication of the diabetes.

No matter what you have learned about the patient's present and past medical history, you need to be aware of certain medical problems that the patient may have forgotten to mention. These conditions might help to explain the current episode or could affect your treatment decisions or those made by ALS or at the hospital. As you conclude the SAMPLE history, ask the patient the following questions:

1. "Have you ever been told that you have a heart condition?"
2. "Have you ever been told that you have asthma, emphysema, or any other problems with your lungs?"
3. "Have you ever been told that you have seizures?"

These three questions will prevent you from missing important, potentially life-threatening cardiac, respiratory, or neurologic conditions. If the patient answers "yes" to any of these three questions, reevaluate the chief complaint in light of this new information. If you have time, return to the history questions to learn more about the nature of the problem.

The Focused Physical Exam

Now that you have questioned the patient about the chief complaint, using OPQRST, and have obtained a thorough present and past medical history, you should perform a focused physical exam (Figure 8-23).

The key to this examination is to examine the areas of the body affected by the chief complaint and associated complaints. Be logical, and investigate problems that you identified during the initial assessment and focused history.

This exam has four priorities:

1. Examine anything associated with an actual or potentially life-threatening condition.
2. Examine anything associated with the patient's chief complaint.
3. Examine anything that has a noticeable abnormality.
4. Evaluate the patient as necessary to obtain baseline information.

Potential or immediate life threats. You should think back to the initial assessment. Did you find any immediately or potentially life-threatening conditions? If so, now is the time to follow up with an exam. Here are some areas to recheck:

- **Abnormal level of consciousness.** Check the head for trauma, and evaluate the breathing and circulation for adequacy.
- **Obstructed airway.** Look inside the mouth and at the back of the throat for foreign bodies, blood, vomitus, or any other substance that might obstruct the airway. Check the neck for signs of abnormality.
- **Inadequate or labored breathing.** Check the airway for obstruction, and evaluate the neck for signs of abnormality. Check the chest for accessory muscle use, and listen to the breath sounds.
- **Inadequate circulation.** Look for blood loss (possibly associated with vomiting), and evaluate the skin color, temperature and condition for signs of inadequate perfusion. Assess the pulse and blood pressure. Check the neck, chest and abdomen for signs of abnormality.

Chief complaint. Once you know that the ABC is stable or stabilized, then examine areas of the body associated with the patient's chief complaint and additional complaints. Remember to carefully assess the following chief complaints, as described previously:

- **Chest pain.** Evaluate the skin color, temperature, and condition, as well as, the pulse, and blood pressure. Look for abnormalities to the chest, and listen to the breath sounds..
- **Shortness of breath.** Check for airway obstruction, as well as abnormalities to the neck and chest. Listen carefully to the breath sounds. Evaluate the skin color, temperature and condition, as well as the pulse, blood pressure, and rate and depth of respirations.
- **Abdominal pain.** Evaluate the skin color, temperature, and condition, as well as the pulse, and blood pressure. Look for abnormalities to the abdomen, and palpate the abdomen to identify any particularly tender areas.
- **Any pain associated with bones or joints.** Evaluate the skin color, temperature and condition, as well as, distal pulses, movement, and sensation.
- **Dizziness.** Evaluate the skin color, temperature and condition, as well as, the pulse, blood pressure, and adequacy of respirations. Monitor the level of consciousness and orientation carefully. Check the head for signs of trauma.

Abnormalities. Next, examine anything that has a noticeable abnormality. Sometimes, during the initial assessment and focused history, you will see something that is obviously abnormal. It may be a cut, a deformed bone, a weakness on one side, abnormal eyes, or some other abnormality. Be sure to ask the patient questions about the abnormality while you are evaluating it. Remember that deformities or abnormalities may be long-term and unrelated to the patient's present condition. For example, a patient who has had a stroke may have a weakness on one side for months after the stroke; it is not a new problem, and it is not likely to be related to the patient's current call for EMS.

Baseline Vital Signs

As you know, baseline vital signs provide useful information about the overall functions of the patient's heart and lungs. Remember that if the patient's condition is stable, you should reassess the vital signs every 15 minutes until you reach the emergency department. If the patient is unstable, you should reassess at a minimum of every 5 minutes, or as often as the situation permits.

Emergency Medical Care and Transport

Your next steps are to provide any additional emergency medical care addressing the chief complaint, associated complaints, and then to provide transport to the emergency department.

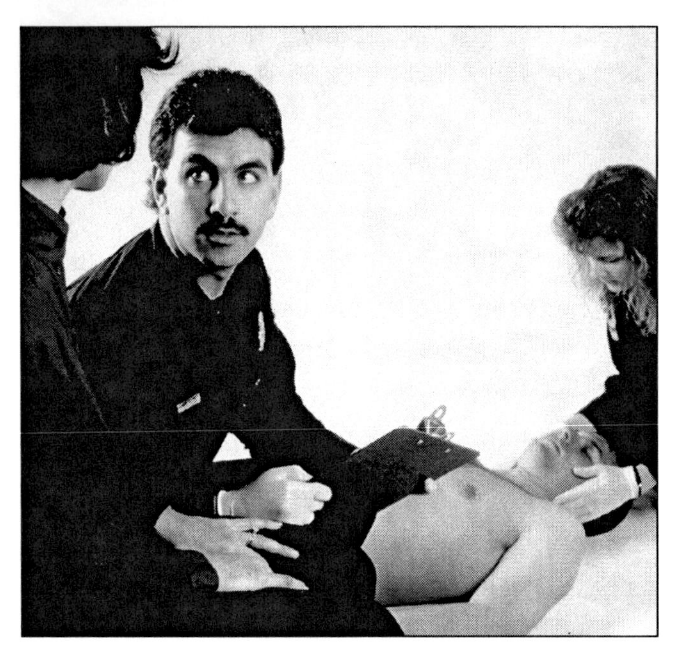

FIGURE 8-24 If the patient is unresponsive, obtain the chief complaint and any other pertinent history from family or bystanders if possible.

Documentation

Documenting your assessment findings helps to identify and track trends in the patient's condition. It also helps hospital staff provide definitive treatment. Your report should include documentation of the following:

- Findings and interventions from the initial assessment
- Findings and interventions from the focused (medical) exam, including pertinent positive and negatives. Findings from the history of present illness, OPQRST.
- Baseline vital signs (respirations, pulse, blood pressure), skin CTC, and pupils)
- SAMPLE history

Assessing the Unresponsive Patient

Sometimes, new EMT-Bs ask how to assess the chief complaint and history of present illness in an unresponsive patient (Figure 8-24). The answer is simple: You cannot.

With unresponsive patients, you will probably never get to that part of the focused history and physical

4

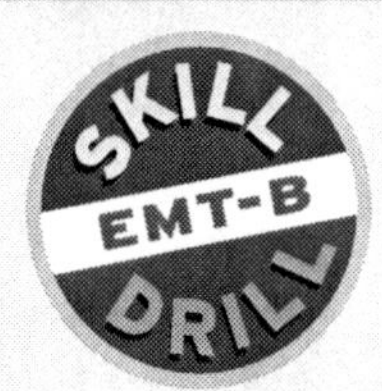

Performing a Rapid Medical Assessment: Unresponsive Patient

Figure 8-25

1

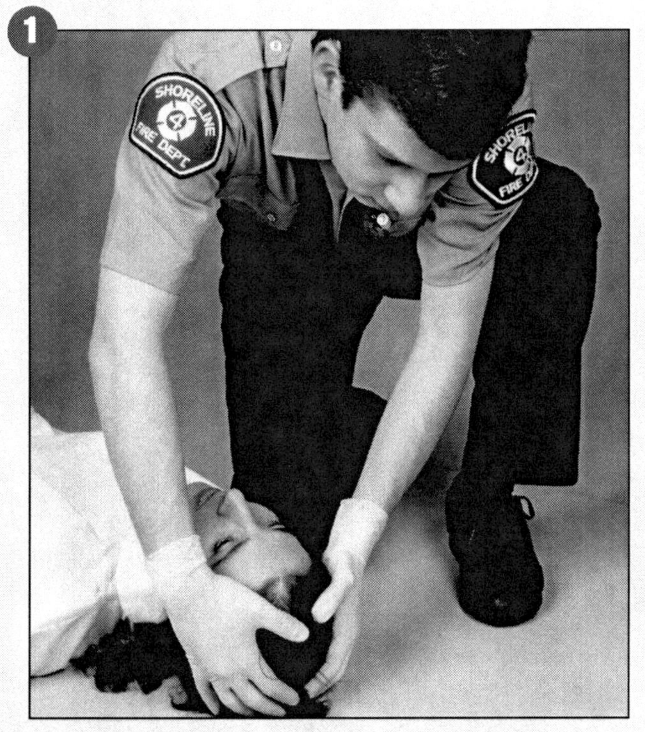

Assess the head for any abnormalities and crepitation.

2

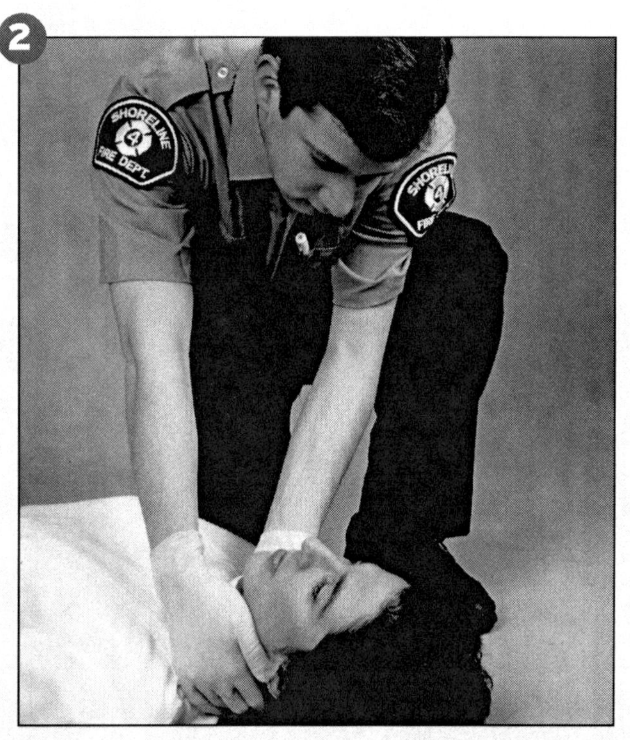

Assess the neck for jugular vein distention, crepitation, and any abnormalities.

3

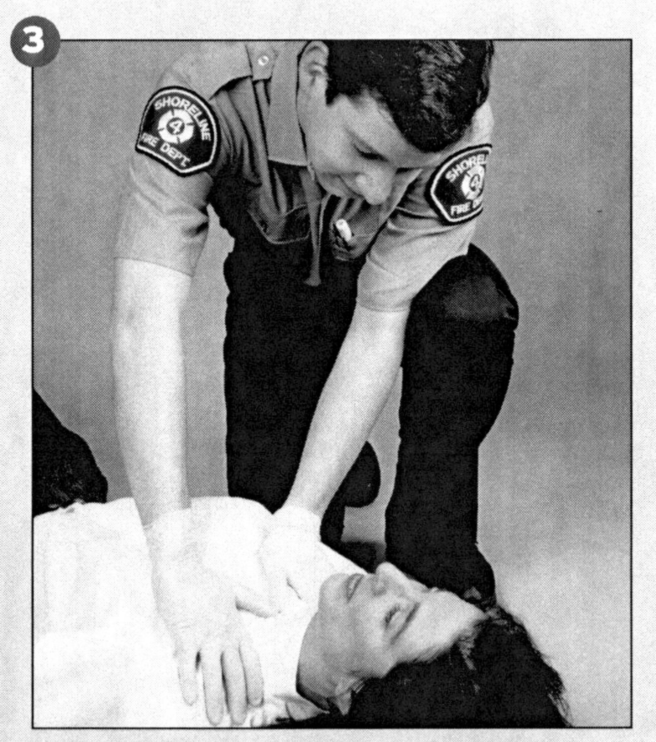

Assess the chest for accessory muscle use, crepitation, and listen to breath sounds.

4

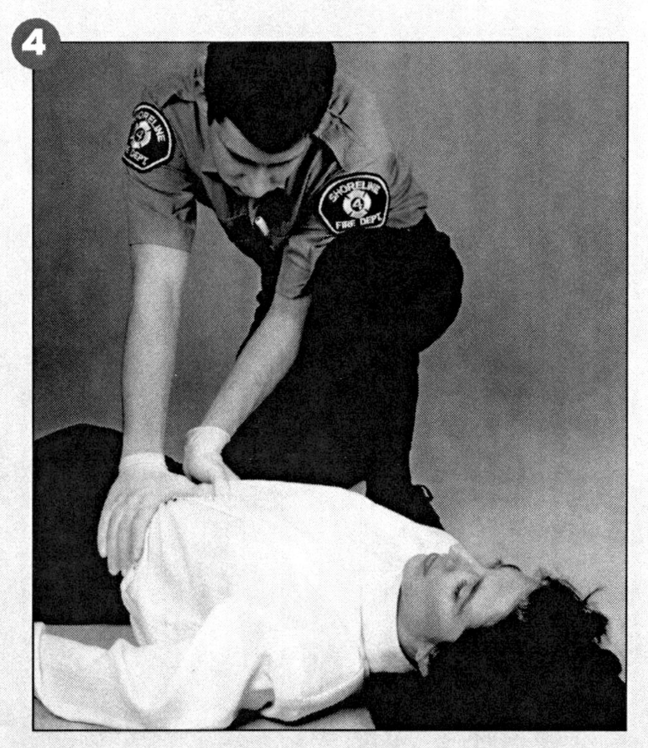

Assess the abdomen for rigidity, distention, pain on palpation, and any other abnormalities.

(Continued)

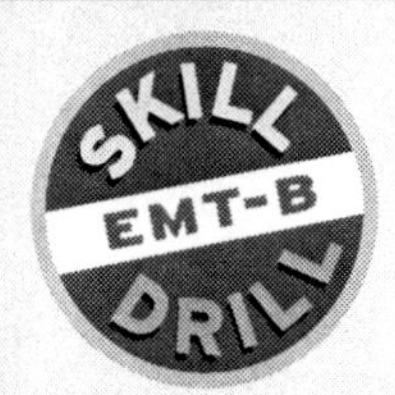

Performing a Rapid Medical Assessment: Unresponsive Patient—cont'd.

Figure 8-25

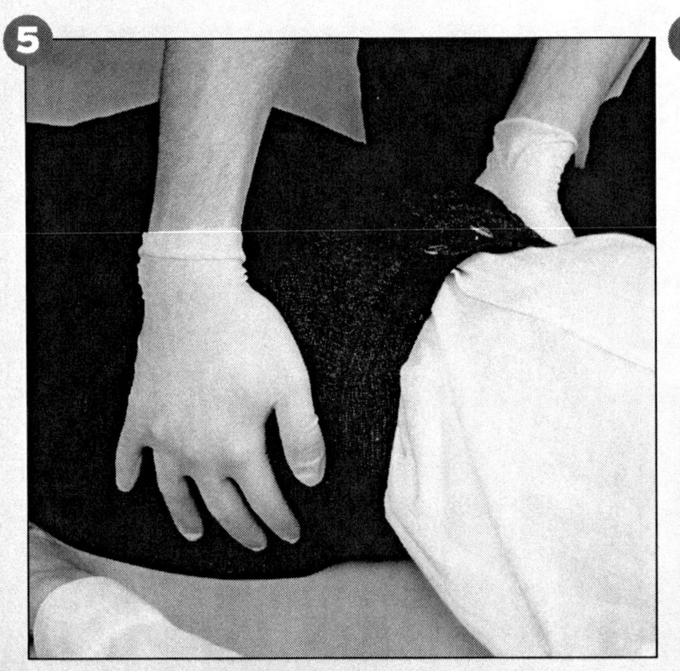

Assess the pelvis for abnormalities.

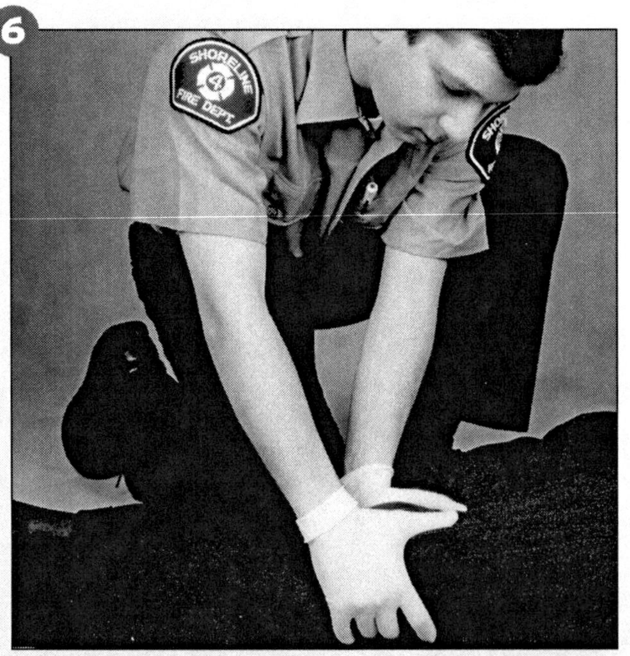

Assess all four extremities for abnormalities and distal pulses, motor and sensory function.

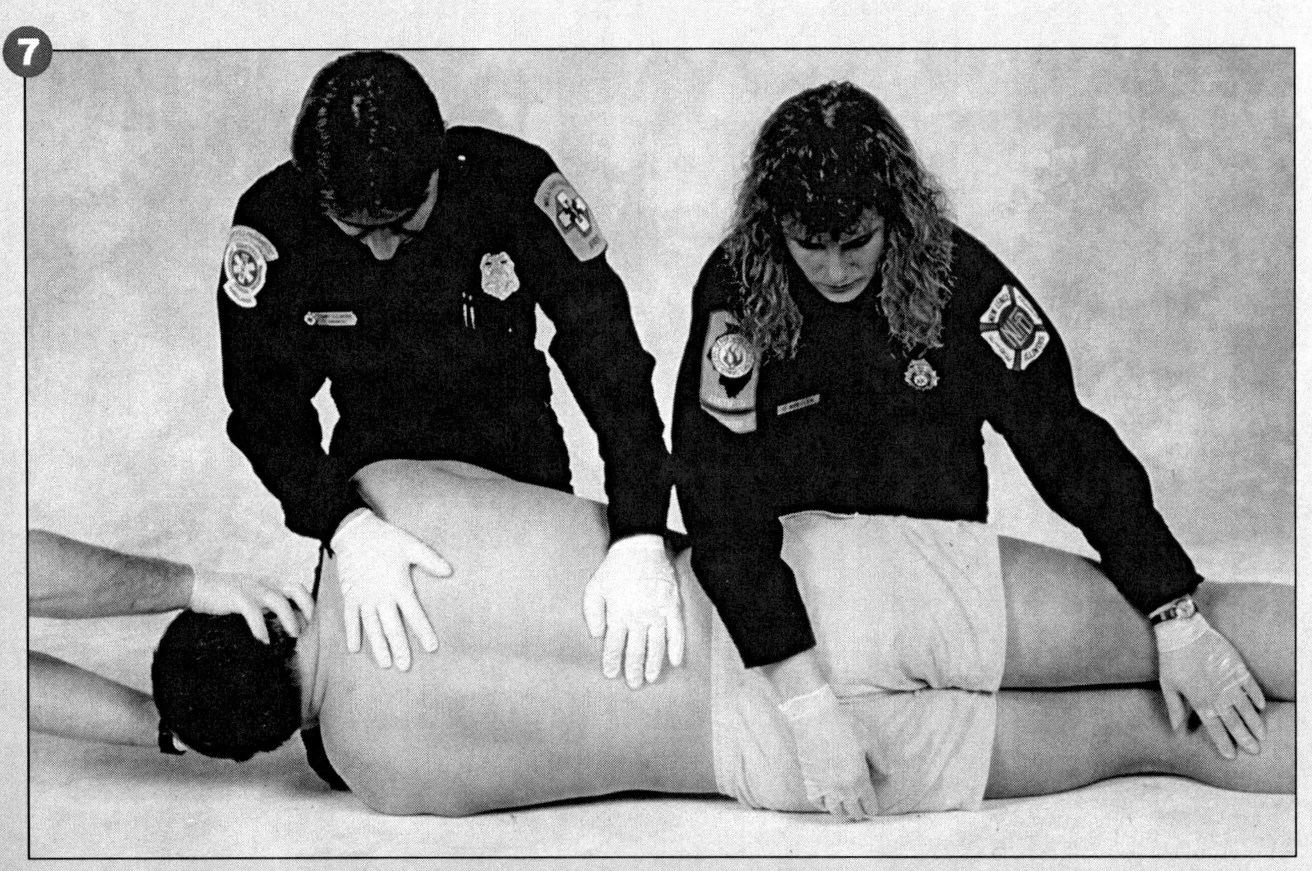

Assess the back for any abnormalities.

4

exam. Instead, you should focus your attention on opening and maintaining the airway, immobilizing the spine if indicated, assisting with ventilations if indicated, administering supplemental oxygen, controlling bleeding, providing CPR if necessary, and providing rapid transport to an appropriate facility. These priorities reflect the importance of the ABCD approach to the initial assessment.

If you have successfully stabilized the ABCD, you ask chief complaint and SAMPLE history questions of a family member or bystander while en route to the hospital. Never delay transport of a critical patient to take a history from family members (or from the patient, for that matter) at the scene.

The Rapid Medical Assessment

Once you have successfully stabilized ABC, you can on any patient who is unconscious, confused, or unable to adequately relate the chief complaint, you should perform a rapid assessment. It is performed in a head-to-toe manner without using the mnemonic "DCAP-BTLS," but it does follow the order of the rapid trauma assessment. The purpose of the rapid medical assessment is to quickly identify existing or potentially life-threatening conditions. Briefly, the sequence of the assessment is as follows (Figure 8-25):

1. Head
2. Neck
3. Chest
4. Abdomen
5. Pelvis
6. Extremities
7. Back

Baseline Vital Signs

Baseline vital signs should be obtained after the rapid medical assessment to provide information for trending. Remember, if the patient's condition is stable (which would not be true for an unresponsive patient), you should reassess the vital signs every 15 minutes until you reach the emergency department. If the patient is unstable, you should reassess at a minimum of every 5 minutes, or as often as the situation permits, looking for trends in the patient's condition.

Emergency Medical Care and Transport

During the focused history and physical exam you will provide the necessary emergency medical care addressing the presenting problems and provide transport to the emergency department. Remember, the patient's spine should be immobilized if you suspect significant trauma or if there is a mechanism of injury that would make you suspect a spinal injury.

Documentation

Documenting your assessment findings helps to identify and track trends in the patient's condition. It also helps hospital staff provide definitive treatment. Your report should include documentation of the following:

- Findings and interventions from the initial assessment
- Findings and interventions from the rapid medical assessment, including pertinent positive and negatives. Findings from the history of present illness, OPQRST, if available.
- Baseline vital signs (respirations, pulse, blood pressure, skin CTC, and pupils)
- SAMPLE history, if available

Detailed Physical Exam

Recall that the assessment process began with anticipation and hazard preparation when you received the dispatch information and performed the scene size-up. Then you performed the initial assessment. You provided treatment of life threats, if identified during the initial assessment. If trauma was a factor in your patient's situation, you also performed spinal stabilization. You followed up on the initial assessment by performing a focused history and physical exam. You also initiated rapid transport procedures if your patient had an obvious life-threatening condition. On the basis of what you learned from the history, you assessed selected areas of the patient's body. You have also taken at least one set of vital signs.

The detailed physical exam is not performed on a patient with a minor injury or minor illness. If the patient is a candidate for the detailed physical exam, you are already enroute to the hospital when you consider performing it. If you are still on the scene, it is because of circumstances beyond your control. The goals of this exam are to further explore problems that were identified during the focused history and physical exam and to possibly identify the cause of complaints that were not identified during the focused history and physical exam.

To achieve these goals, you must simply ask and answer one question: "What additional problems can be identified through a detailed physical exam?" The detailed physical exam will provide you with more information about the nature of the patient's problem. Depending on what is learned, you should be prepared to do the following:

- Return to the initial assessment if a potentially life-threatening condition is identified. (This is unlikely this late in the exam, but it is always possible. Remember, stay focused on the ABC.)
- Modify any treatment that is underway on the basis of any new information.
- Provide treatment for problems that were identified during the exam.

5

Goals of the Detailed Physical Exam

The detailed physical exam is a more in-depth examination that builds on the focused physical exam. The patient and the particular injury will determine the need for this exam. Many of your patients will not receive a detailed physical exam, either because it will be irrelevant or unnecessary or because it is not possible given the time constraints.

Most patients have isolated problems that can be adequately evaluated earlier in the assessment process. You will identify the problem and treat it, making a more detailed physical exam of the entire body unnecessary. If you do perform a detailed physical exam in patients, it will be to further explore what you learned during the focused history and physical exam.

Some patients will have life-threatening conditions that were identified during the initial assessment. You may spend all of your time with these patients, stabilizing ABC, which means you may never have a chance to perform a detailed physical exam.

You will perform a detailed exam only on patients who are victims of significant mechanism of injury or patients with problems that cannot be adequately identified earlier in the patient assessment process. Regardless of the exact situation, the detailed physical exam should be performed enroute to the hospital, since you could literally spend hours on the scene trying to identify all of the patient's problems.

Sequence of the Detailed Physical Exam

Here, organized by body region, are some additional assessments that you might want to perform during the detailed exam. As you evaluate each region, visualize and palpate to find evidence of signs of injury, again using the mnemonic "DCAP-BTLS" (Figure 8-26). Table 8-14 lists the components of the detailed physical exam.

Head, Neck, and Cervical Spine

A more detailed exam of these areas could include a careful check of the head, face, scalp, ears, eyes, nose, and mouth for abrasions, lacerations, and contusions. Examine the eyes and eyelids, checking for redness and

PATIENT ASSESSMENT FLOWCHART

Detailed Physical Exam

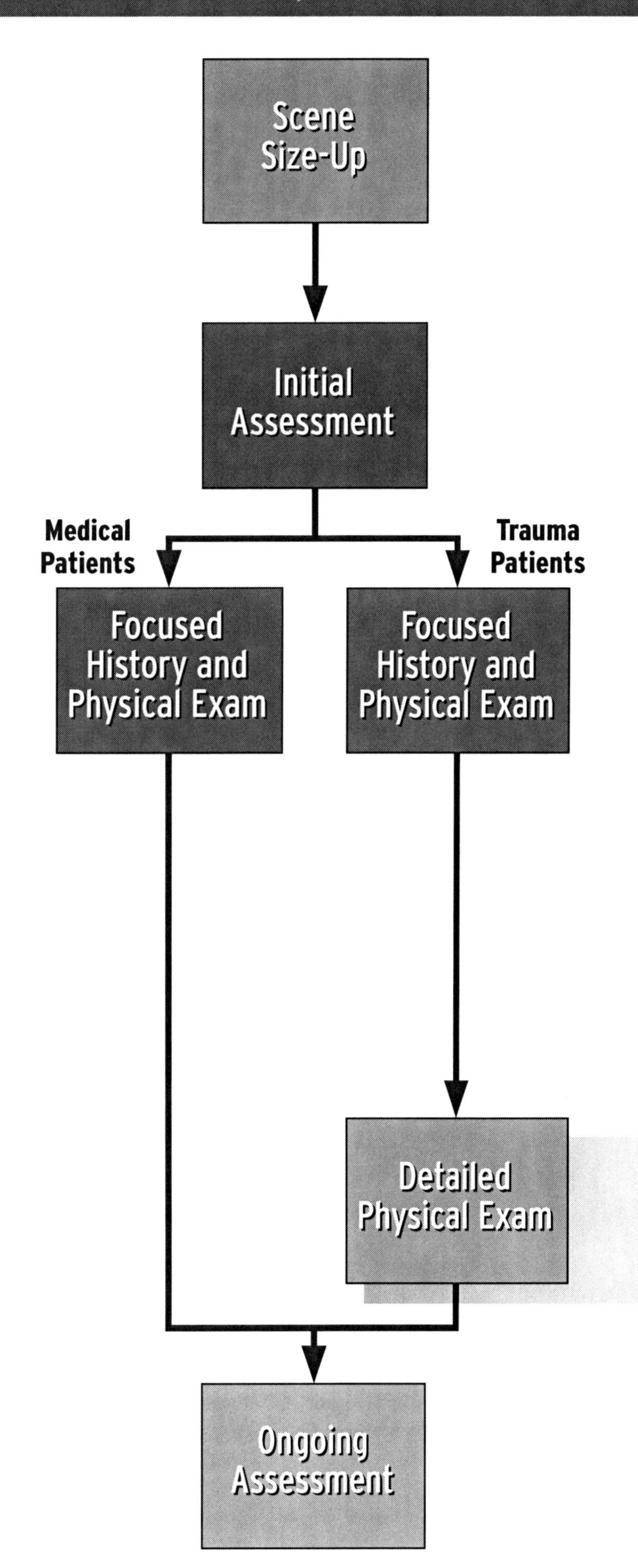

5

TABLE 8-14 Components of the Detailed Physical Exam

As you inspect and palpate, look and/or feel for the following examples of injuries or signs of injuries: DCAP-BTLS

Assess	Look For	Assess	Look For
Head	• DCAP-BTLS	**Chest**	• DCAP-BTLS • Crepitus • Paradoxical motion • Breath sounds
Face	• DCAP-BTLS	**Abdomen**	• DCAP-BTLS • Firmness • Softness • Tenderness • Distention
Ears	• DCAP-BTLS • Drainage • Bruising or discoloration (Battle's sign)	**Pelvis**	• DCAP-BTLS • Pain • Tenderness • Instability • Crepitus
Eyes	• DCAP-BTLS • Redness • Contact lenses • Equal and reactive pupils • Fluid and drainage • Foreign objects • Bruising or discoloration (raccoon eyes)	**Extremities**	• DCAP-BTLS • Distal circulation • Sensation • Movement
Nose	• DCAP-BTLS • Drainage • Bleeding	**Back**	• DCAP-BTLS (roll with spinal precautions before securing to a long backboard)
Mouth	• DCAP-BTLS • Broken or missing teeth or a foreign object • Obstructions • Swollen or lacerated tongue • Unusual breath odors • Discoloration		
Neck	• DCAP-BTLS • Subcutaneous emphysema • Jugular vein distention • Crepitus		

for contact lenses. Use a penlight to check whether the pupils are equal and reactive, and look for any fluid drainage or blood, particularly around the ears and nose. Also check for foreign objects and/or blood in the anterior chamber of the eye. Look for bruising or discoloration around the eyes (raccoon eyes) or behind the ears (Battle's sign); these signs may be associated with head trauma.

Next, palpate gently but firmly around the face, scalp, eyes, ears, and nose for tenderness, deformity, or instability. Tenderness or abnormal movement of bones often signals a serious injury and may cause upper airway obstruction. Monitor the airway carefully in these patients. Look and feel inside the mouth next. Loose or broken teeth or a foreign object may block the airway. Remember, be cautious when inserting your fingers into a patient's mouth. It's much safer if a bite block is used. You should also look for lacerations, swelling, bleeding, and any discoloration in the mouth and the tongue.

SKILL DRILL EMT-B

Performing the Detailed Physical Exam

Figure 8-26

1

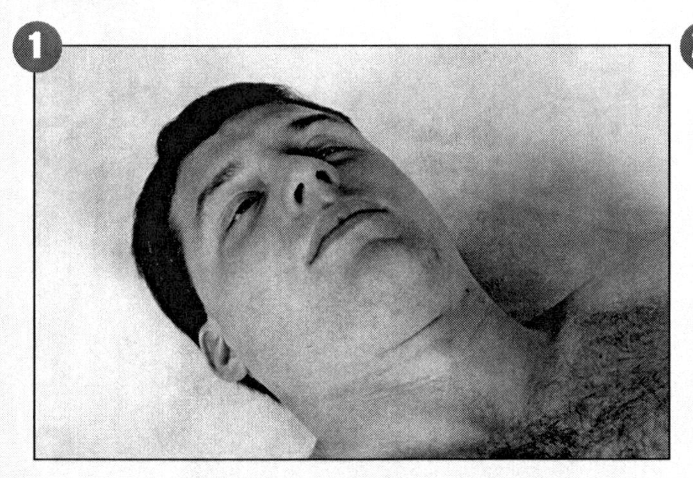

Look at the face for obvious lacerations, bruises, or deformities.

2

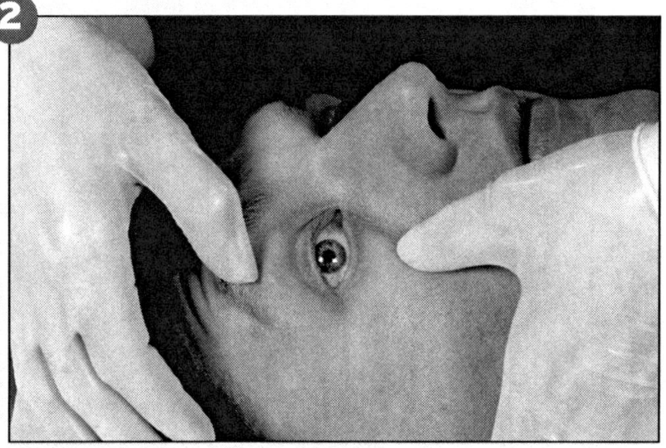

Inspect the area around the eyes and eyelids.

3

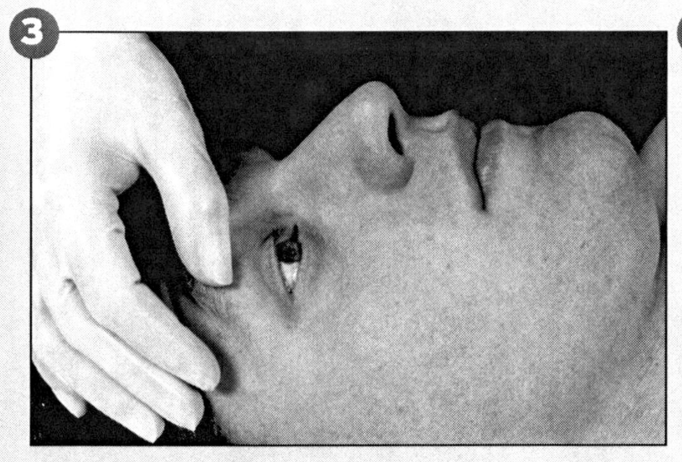

Examine the eyes for redness and for contact lenses. Assess the pupils using a penlight.

4

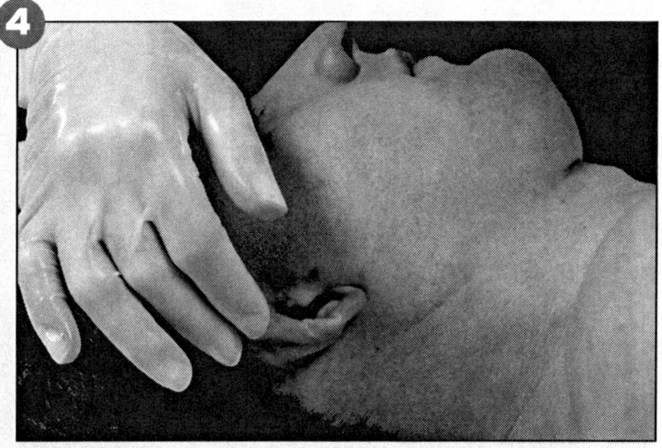

Pull the patient's ear forward to assess for bruising (Battle's sign).

5

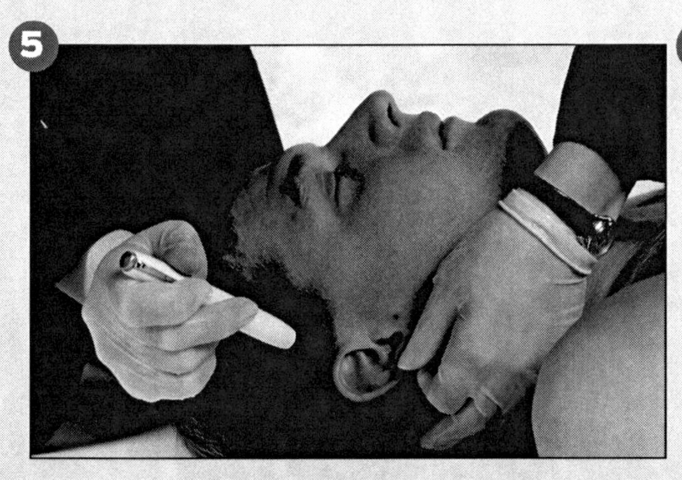

Use the penlight to look for drainage or blood in the ears.

6

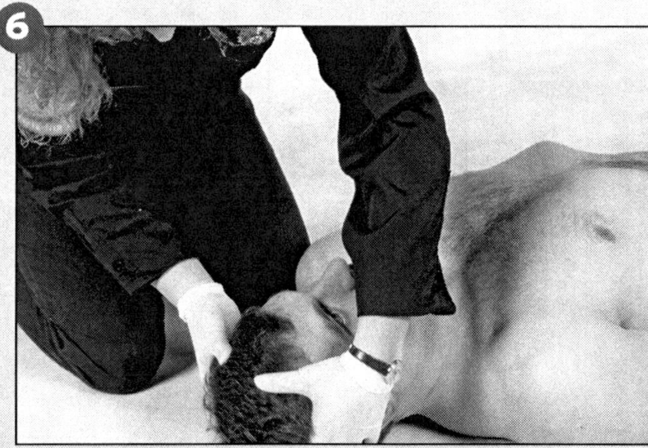

Look for bruising and lacerations about the head. Palpate for tenderness, depressions of the skull, and deformities.

(Continued)

5

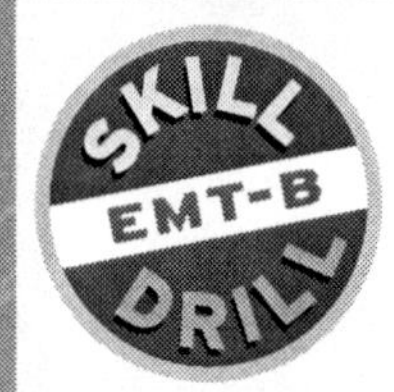

Performing the Detailed Physical Exam—cont'd.

Figure 8-26

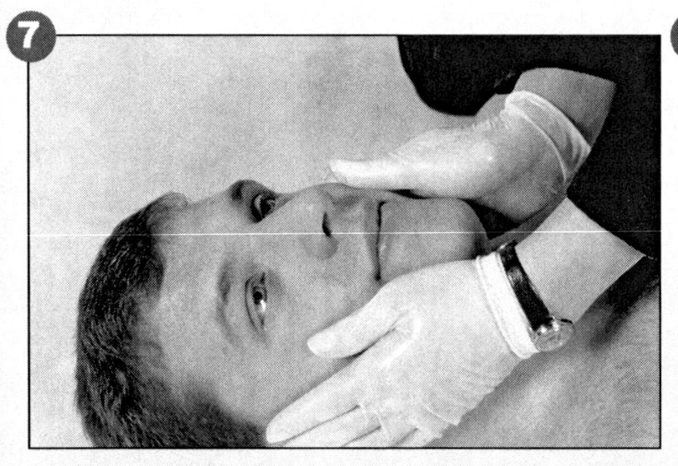

Palpate the zygomas (cheek bones) for tenderness or instability.

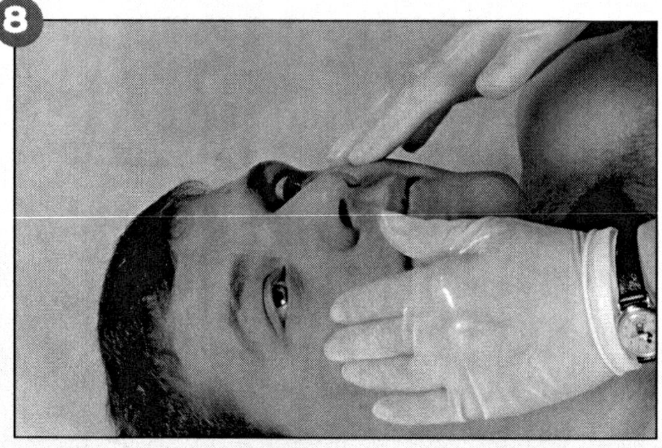

Palpate the maxillae (upper jaw).

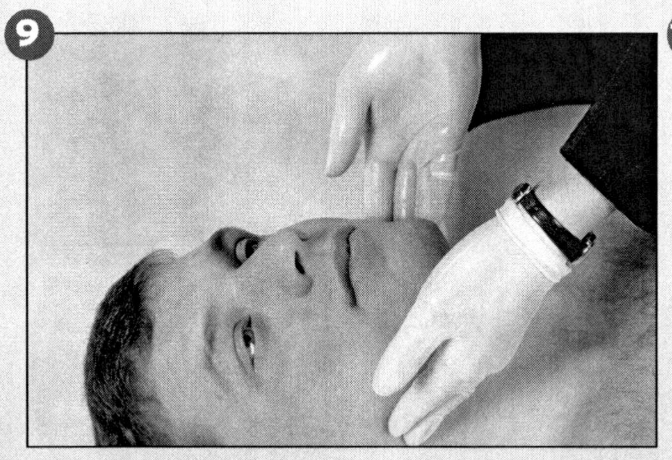

Palpate the mandible (lower jaw).

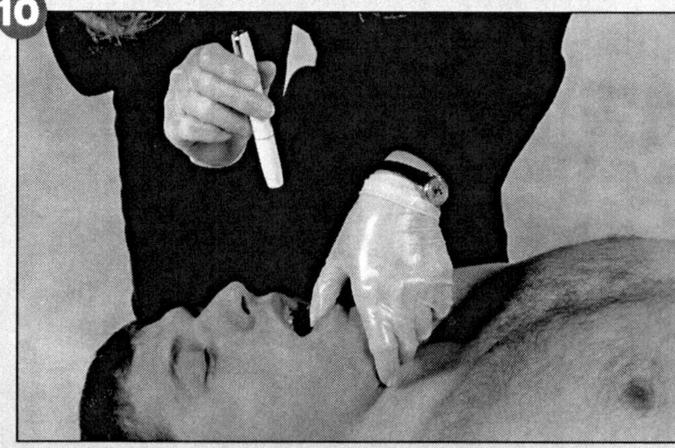

Assess the mouth for cyanosis, foreign bodies (including loose teeth or dentures), bleeding, lacerations, or deformities.

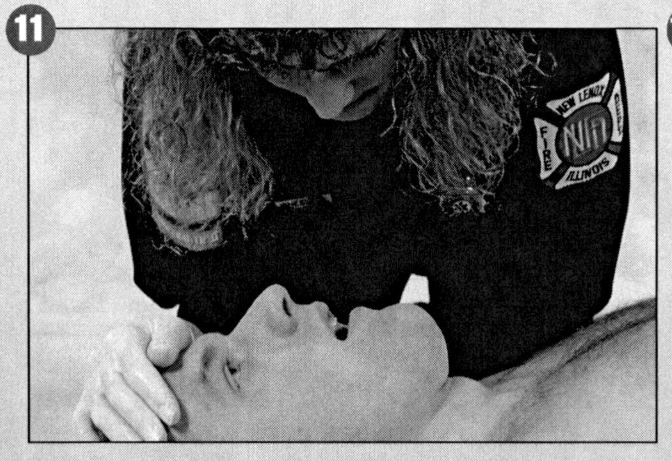

Check for unusual odors on the patient's breath.

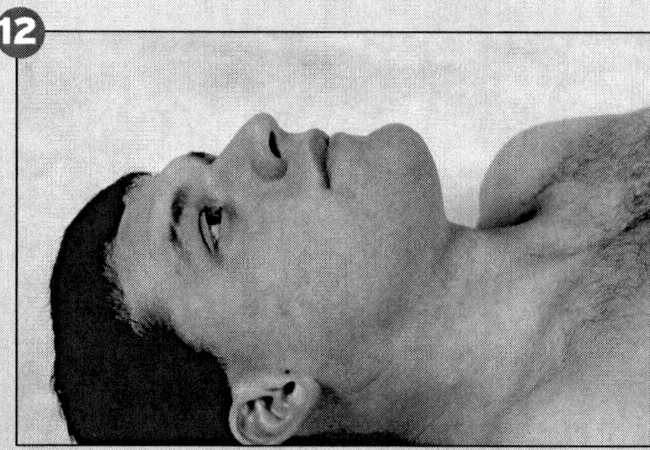

Look at the neck for obvious lacerations, bruises, and deformities.

13

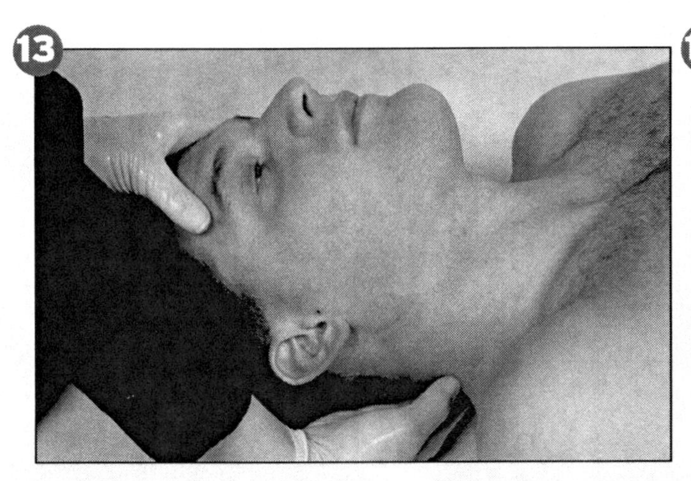

If the cervical collar does not interfere, palpate the front and the back of the neck for tenderness

14

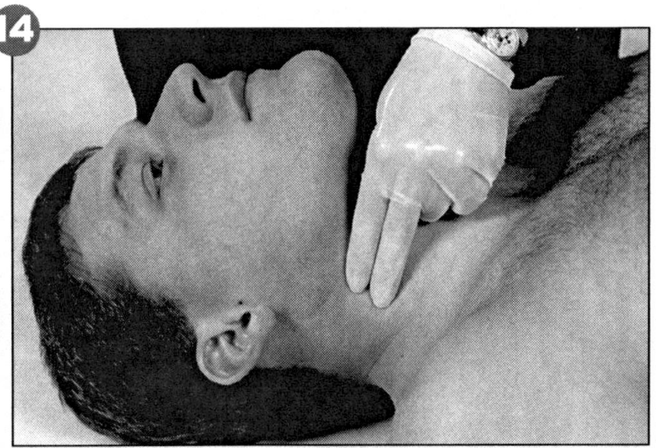

Look for distended jugular veins. Note that distended neck veins are not necessarily significant in a patient who is lying down.

15

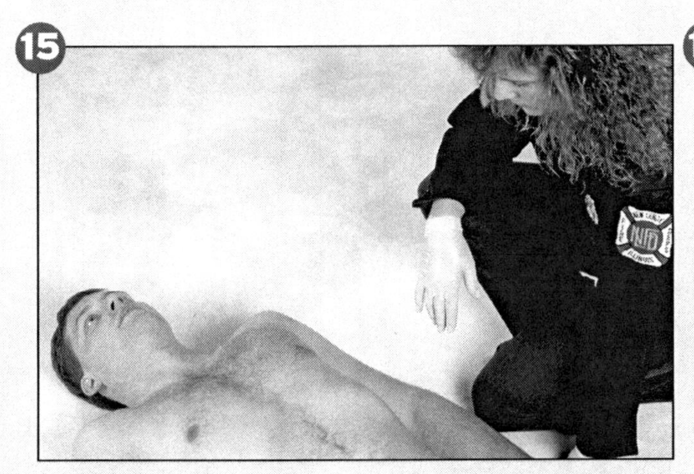

Look at the chest for obvious signs of injury before you begin palpation. Be sure to watch for movement of the chest with respirations.

16

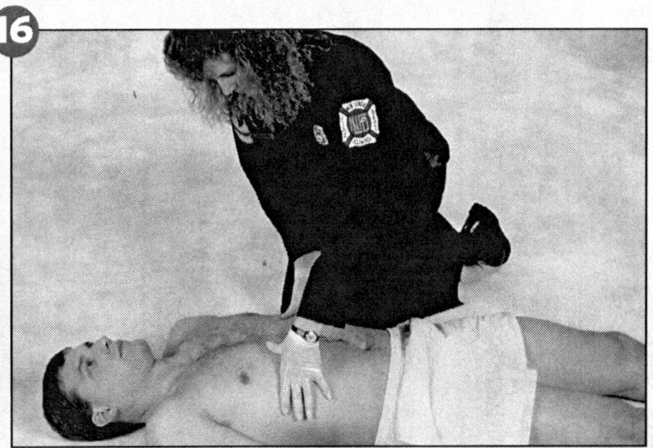

Gently palpate over the ribs to elicit tenderness. Avoid pressing over obvious bruises or fractures.

17

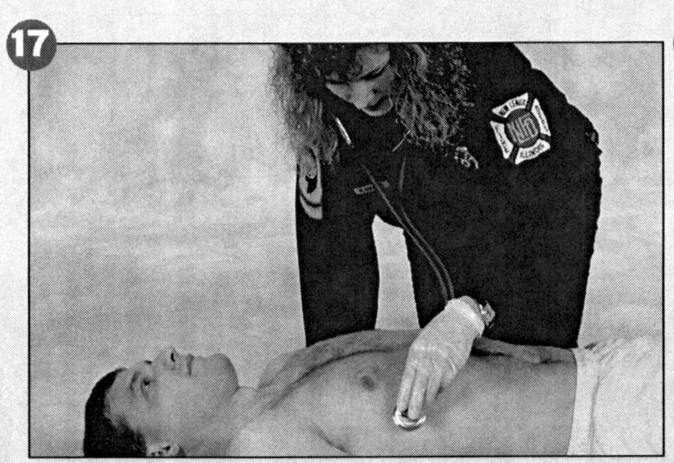

Listen for breath sounds over the midaxillary and midclavicular lines.

18

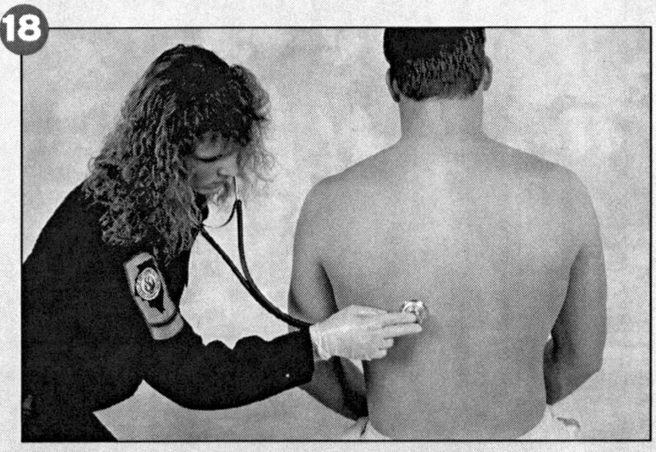

Listen also at the bases and apices of the lungs.

(Continued)

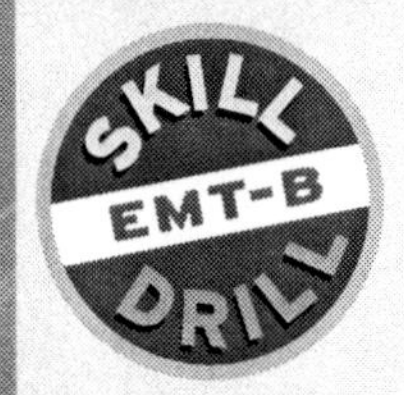

Performing the Detailed Physical Exam—cont'd.

Figure 8-26

19

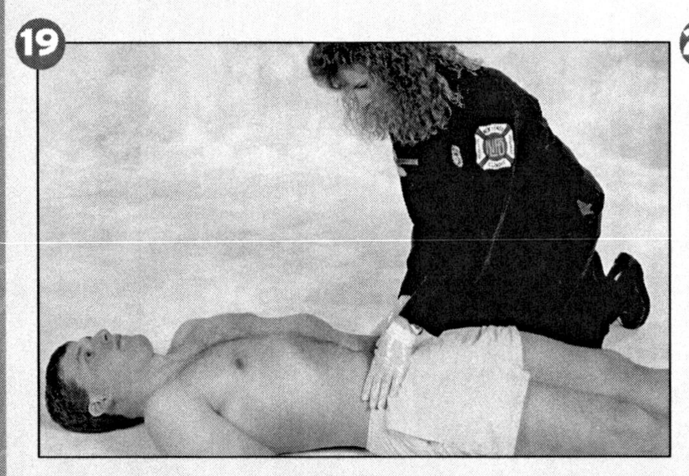

Look at the abdomen and pelvis for obvious lacerations, bruises, and deformities.

20

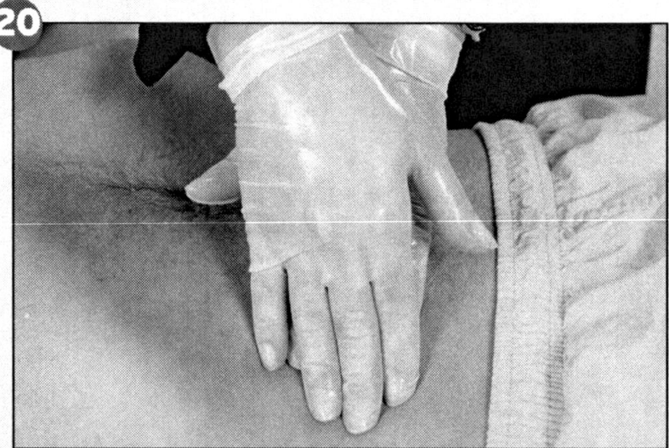

Gently palpate the abdomen for tenderness. If the abdomen is unusually tense, you should describe the abdomen as rigid.

21

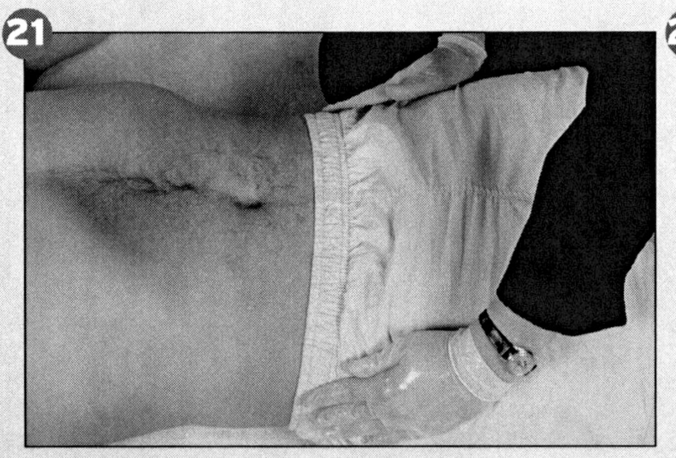

Gently compress the pelvis from the sides to assess for tenderness.

22

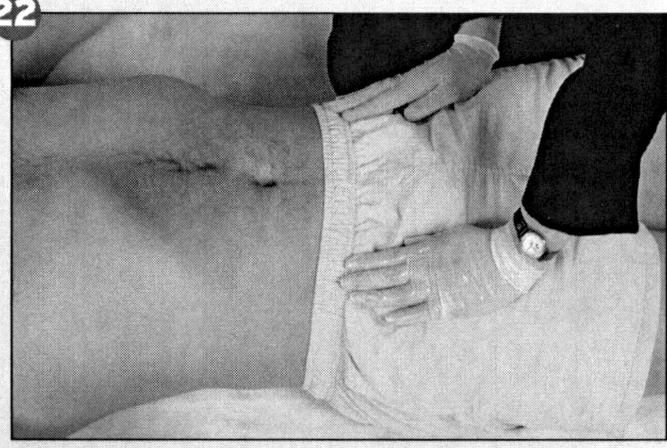

Gently press the iliac crests to elicit instability, tenderness, or crepitation.

23

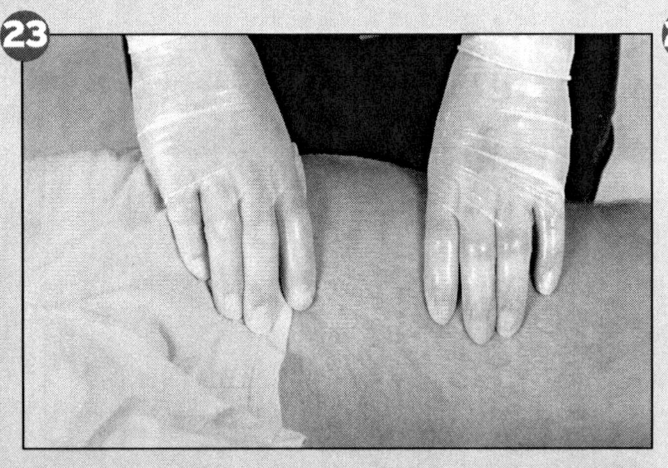

Inspect all four extremities for lacerations, bruises, swelling, and deformities. Also assess distal circulation, sensation, and movement in all extremities.

24

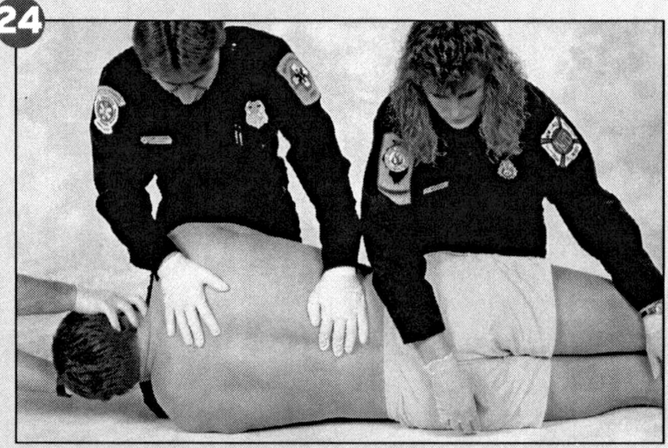

Remember, if the patient was a victim of significant mechanism of injury, then you have already performed spinal immobilization, making assessment of the back for tenderness or deformities impossible.

Smell the patient's breath. Any unusual odors, such as a strong alcohol odor or fruity breath odor, should be reported and recorded.

Palpation of the front and back of the neck for tenderness and deformity will not be possible if the patient is already immobilized. But you can look for pronounced or distended jugular veins. This can be normal in a patient who is lying down; however, their presence in the patient who is sitting up may suggest some type of damage to the heart.

Chest

Throughout the patient assessment process, you should monitor the patient's breathing. Evaluate the movement of the chest wall during breathing. Perform a more detailed evaluation of the patient's breath sounds. Listening at the apices, at the midclavicular lines bilaterally, at the bases, and at the midaxillary lines bilaterally, check for the specific sounds of breathing. You may be able to identify one of the following:

- Normal breath sounds. These are clear and quiet on both inspiration and expiration.
- Wheezing breath sounds. These suggest an obstruction of the lower airways. Wheezing is a high-pitched squeal that is most prominent on expiration.
- Wet breath sounds. These may indicate cardiac failure. A moist crackling, usually on both inspiration and expiration is called rales, or crackles.
- Congested breath sounds. These may suggest the presence of mucus in the lungs. Expect to hear a low-pitched, noisy sound that is most prominent on expiration. This sound may be referred to as rhonchi, or "low wheezing." The patient often reports a productive cough associated with this sound.
- A crowing sound. This is often heard without a stethoscope and may indicate that the patient has an airway obstruction in the neck or upper part of the chest. Expect to hear a brassy, crowing sound that is most prominent on expiration. This sound may be referred to as stridor.

Abdomen

During the detailed physical exam, you may perform a more complete examination of the abdomen. As you feel all around the abdomen, use the terms firm, soft, tender, or distended (swollen) to report your findings. Some patients may tense the abdomen as you feel it. This reaction may be caused by a ticklish or overly sensitive patient or may be a condition known as guarding, which is often associated with damage to organs within the abdomen.

Pelvis

If you have not previously identified any abnormality, recheck the pelvis to identify pain, tenderness, instability, and crepitus; all may indicate a fractured pelvis and the potential for shock.

Extremities

If you have not already done so, you should carefully evaluate the extremities for any signs of trauma, again using the DCAP-BTLS method. You should also evaluate the distal circulation, sensation, and movement. If you have already identified an injury, regular evaluation of the circulation, sensation, and movement below the injury will allow you to be sure that the injury has not compromised circulation.

Back

During the rapid assessment, you should have visualized and palpated the patient's back for signs of trauma, especially near the spine. Remember, the detailed physical exam is performed while enroute to the hospital, typically on a patient who is a victim of significant mechanism of injury. In that case, the patient is already immobilized to a long backboard, and hence, inspection and palpation of the back is impossible.

Assess Baseline Vital Signs

Sometimes, you will be so busy establishing and maintaining the ABC that you will not have a chance to get the patient's vital signs. That is as it should be. Nothing should take priority over the airway, breathing, and circulation. However, whenever possible, it is important to get a set of baseline vitals at some time during your patient encounter. If you have not assessed the vital signs, now is the time.

Ongoing Assessment

Unlike the detailed physical exam, ongoing assessment is performed on all patients during transport. Its purpose is to ask and answer the following questions:

- Is treatment improving the patient's condition?
- Has an already identified problem gotten better? Worse?
- What is the nature of any newly identified problems?

The ongoing assessment helps you to monitor changes in the patient's condition. If the changes are improvements, simply continue whatever treatment you are providing. However, in some instances, the patient's condition will become worse. When this happens, you should be prepared to modify treatment as appropriate and then begin new treatment on the basis of the problem identified.

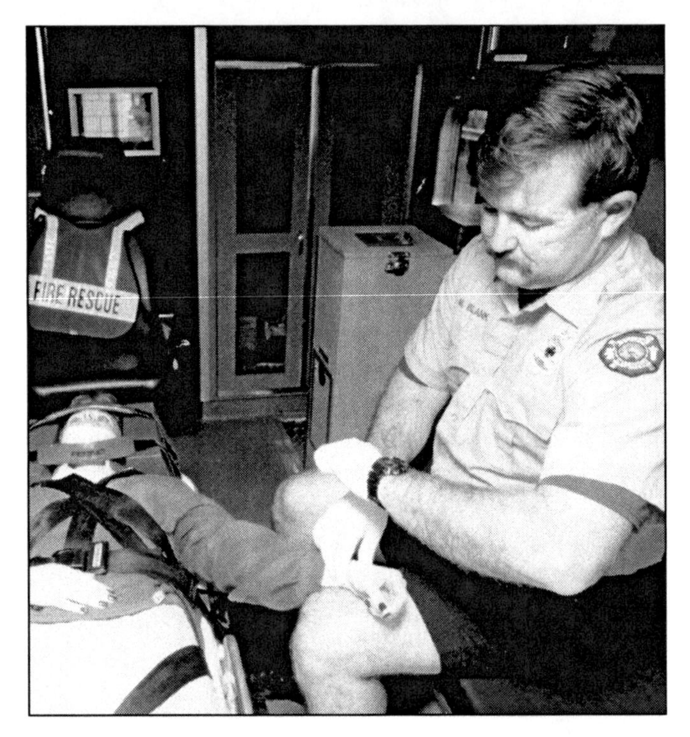

FIGURE 8-27 During the ongoing assessment, repeat your initial assessment, recheck vital signs, and recheck interventions every 5 minutes if the patient is unstable and every 15 minutes if the patient is stable.

Steps of the Ongoing Assessment

The procedure for the ongoing assessment is simply to repeat the initial assessment and the focused assessment and to check the intervention steps that pertain to the problems you are treating. These steps should be repeated and recorded every 15 minutes for a stable patient and every 5 minutes for an unstable patient (Figure 8-27). Remember to use your judgment when timing the ongoing assessments. Some patients may require more frequent assessments.

The steps of the ongoing assessment are as follows:

1. Repeat the initial assessment.
   - Reassess the general impression.
   - Reassess mental status.
   - Maintain an open airway.
   - Monitor the patient's breathing.
   - Reassess pulse rate and quality.
   - Monitor skin color, temperature, and condition (skin CTC).
   - Reestablish patient priorities.
2. Reassess and record vital signs.
3. Repeat your focused assessment regarding patient complaint or injuries, including questions about the patient's history.
4. Check interventions.
   - Ensure adequacy of oxygen delivery/artificial ventilation.
   - Ensure management of bleeding.
   - Ensure adequacy of other interventions.

Repeat the Initial Assessment

The first step is to repeat the initial assessment. If you have been treating the ABC, you need to continue monitoring these essential functions. It is particularly important to reassess mental status; changes can be initially subtle and then rapid.

Reevaluate any problems that you have been treating. Reassess the patient's skin color, wound, or anything for which you have begun treatment. If the patient's condition remains stable, great. But, you may discover a need to change a dressing, tighten a strap, or turn up the oxygen. Do it now.

Reassess and Record Vital Signs

Be sure that the patient's vital signs have not changed. Record these so that your documentation is accurate and complete. If the vital signs have changed, evaluate what may have happened and what you should do about it.

PATIENT ASSESSMENT FLOWCHART

Ongoing Assessment

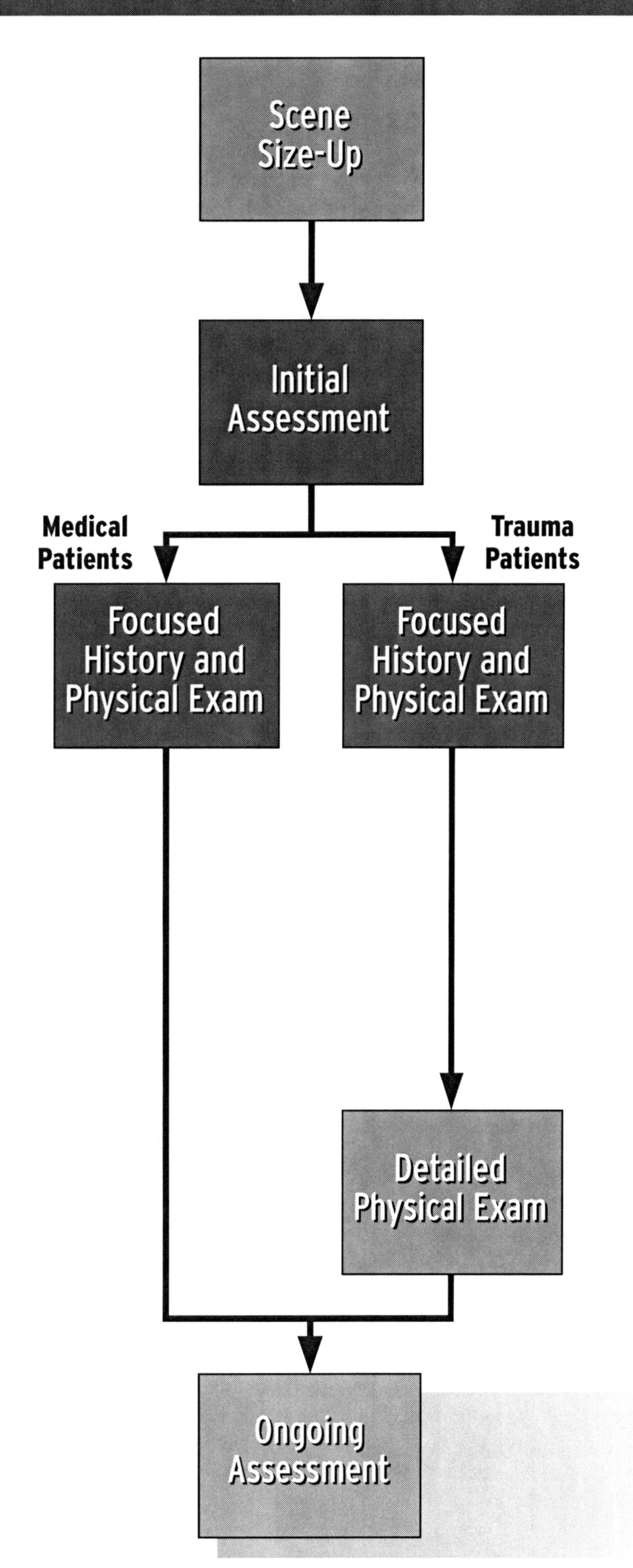

6

becoming an expert

You may notice at times that experienced EMT-Bs and paramedics seem to have a "sixth sense" when it comes to some patients. They seem to be able to recognize severe problems even before they have completed their initial assessment. This clinical intuition is one of the hallmarks of the expert EMT that you can develop as you progress through your career—if you pay attention and work at it.

The aspects of clinical intuition include the following:

- **The ability to recognize patterns.** Intuitive EMTs immediately recognize clinical patterns that they have seen before. For example, you may immediately recognize that a pale, diaphoretic patient looks like another patient you have seen in severe shock.
- **Common sense understanding.** Experienced, intuitive EMTs who use their knowledge and experience also use common sense in their assessment and treatment. For instance, they refrain from starting CPR on a responsive patient even though they cannot feel a pulse.
- **The ability to sense what is important.** Good EMTs know how to track problems that are truly important. They avoid the tendency to get lost in unimportant problems and stay focused on the ones that truly matter. For instance, a forehead laceration will not distract them from the serious cardiac problem that caused a fall.
- Deliberate rationally. Good EMTs use their intuition to help them make decisions, but they always temper it by asking, "What if I'm wrong?" For example, a patient who was in a serious motor vehicle accident but has no complaints and appears normal is probably fine. An experienced EMT-B might believe that the patient has no serious injuries and probably does not require spinal immobilization. However, the answer to the question "What if I'm wrong?" could be "Disastrous: permanent spinal cord injury and paralysis." The experienced EMT-B decides to immobilize.

How can you improve your own intuitive powers? First, you need some experience. The truth is that you will not become intuitive until you have been involved in patient care for some time and have evaluated and treated a number of patients.

By following a systematic approach to patient assessment, using your intuition and common sense, and really listening to the patient, you will learn to make good decisions about the treatment and transport of the many patients you will care for in your career.

Repeat Focused Assessment

As you transport your patient, remember to ask the patient about the chief complaint. Is the chest pain getting better or worse? Is leg pain improving with treatment or staying about the same? If you asked the patient to rate symptoms on a 1 to 10 scale, ask for another rating. Remember that this is the reason the patient called 9-1-1.

Check Interventions

Reevaluate any interventions you started. Take a moment to make certain that the oxygen is still flowing, that the backboard straps are still tight, that the bleeding has been controlled, and that the airway is still open. Things often change in the uncontrolled prehospital environment, so this is a good time to be sure that your treatments are still "working" the way you expect.

prep kit

ready for review

The assessment process begins with evaluation of the dispatch information, which often includes the nature of the call and an early report on the chief complaint. The dispatch information may also provide clues to potential hazards to be found on the scene.

The scene size-up identifies real or potential hazards. The patient should not be approached until these hazards have been dealt with in a way that eliminates or minimizes risk to both the EMTs and the patient(s).

The initial assessment is performed on all patients. It identifies any life-threatening conditions to the airway, breathing, and circulation. Any abnormalities that are found must be treated before moving to the next step of the assessment.

The focused history and physical exam are performed on all patients once their ABC is stabilized. The focused history and physical exam identify potentially life-threatening conditions and help you to identify and explore the patient's chief complaint. In most cases, the focused history and physical exam will provide adequate information to enable you to initiate treatment.

As part of the focused history and physical exam, the rapid trauma assessment or rapid medical assessment, is performed quickly on any patient who is unconscious or unable to articulate the nature of the problem to identify injuries or illnesses. When abnormalities are found, they should be prioritized and treated as appropriate.

The detailed physical exam is performed on a select group of patients. It helps you to further understand problems that were identified during the focused exam and may also be used to evaluate problems that cannot be identified using the focused exam. The detailed physical exam should be performed en route to the hospital.

The ongoing assessment is performed on all patients. It gives you an opportunity to re-evaluate problems that are being treated and to recheck treatments to be sure that they are still being delivered correctly. Information from the ongoing assessment may be used to change treatment plans.

As you can see, the assessment process is both systematic and dynamic. All patients will be evaluated by using these same steps. However, because of the ability of the focused history and physical exam to center your actions on the major problems, each of your assessments will be slightly different, depending on the needs of the patient. The result will be a process that will enable you to quickly identify and treat the needs of all patients, both medical and traumatic, in a way that meets their unique needs.

Patient Assessment Process

Trauma Patient with a Significant Mechanism of Injury	Trauma Patient with No Significant Mechanism of Injury	Medical Patient Who Is Responsive	Medical Patient Who Is Not Responsive
Scene Size-Up			
Initial Assessment			
Focused History/Physical Exam*			
• Reconsider mechanism of injury	• Assess chief complaint	• Assess chief complaint	• Rapid medical assessment
• Rapid trauma assessment	• Focused assessment of area of complaint	• O-P-Q-R-S-T	• Baseline vital signs
• Baseline vital signs	• Baseline vital signs	• Focused physical exam	• SAMPLE history (from family or bystanders)
• SAMPLE history	• SAMPLE history	• Baseline vital signs	
Detailed Physical Exam			
• Area by area exam*			• Area by area exam*
On-Going Assessment*			

* If appropriate

prep kit

vital vocabulary

www.emtb.com

accessory muscles The secondary muscles of respiration.

AVPU A method of assessing a patient's level of consciousness by determining whether a patient is awake and alert, responsive to verbal stimulus or pain, or unresponsive; used principally in the initial assessment.

blunt trauma A mechanism of injury in which force occurs over a broad area and the skin is not usually broken.

body substance isolation (BSI) An infection control concept and practice that assumes that all body fluids are potentially infectious.

breath sounds An indication of air movement in the lungs.

capillary refill A test that evaluates the function of the circulatory system at the distal points in the body.

chief complaint The reason a patient called for help. Also, the patient's response to general questions such as "What's wrong?" or "What happened?"

coagulate Formation of clots to plug openings in injured blood vessels and stop blood flow.

conjunctiva The delicate membrane that lines the eyelids and covers the exposed surface of the eye.

crepitus A grating or grinding sensation caused by fractured bone ends or joints rubbing together. Also air bubbles under the skin, giving the skin a crinkly feeling.

cyanosis Blueish-gray skin color that is caused by reduced oxygen levels in the blood.

DCAP-BTLS A mnemonic for assessment in which each area of the body is evaluated for Deformities, Contusions, Abrasions, Punctures/Penetrations, Burns, Tenderness, Lacerations, and Swelling.

detailed physical exam The part of the assessment process in which a detailed area-by-area exam is performed on patients whose problems cannot be readily identified or when more specific information about problems identified in the focused history and physical exam is necessary.

diffuse pain Pain that is not identified as being specific to a single location.

entrance wound The area of the body where a penetrating trauma occurs. In knife or gunshot wounds, this would be the area where the bullet or blade entered. Also seen in serious electrical injuries.

exit wound The area of the body where a penetrating trauma exited. In gunshot wounds, this would be the area where the bullet exited.

focal pain Pain that is easily identified as being specific to a single location.

focused history and physical exam The part of the assessment process in which the patient's major complaints or any problems that are immediately evident are further and more specifically evaluated.

frostbite Damage to tissues as the result of exposure to cold; frozen or partially frozen body parts.

general impression The overall initial impression that determines the priority for patient care. It is based on the patient's surroundings, the mechanism of injury, or the patient's chief complaint.

Golden hour The period of time during which treatment of a patient in shock or with traumatic injuries is most critical. This period of time is generally thought to be the first 60 minutes after injury.

guarding Involuntary muscle contraction of the abdominal wall in an effort to protect the inflamed abdomen.

hypothermia A condition in which the internal body temperature falls below 95°F (35°C) after exposure to a cold environment.

initial assessment The part of the assessment process that helps you to identify any immediately or potentially life-threatening conditions so that you can initiate lifesaving care.

jaundice A yellow skin color that is seen in patients with liver disease or dysfunction.

mechanism of injury The way in which traumatic injuries occur; the forces that act on the body to cause damage.

nasal flaring Flaring out of the nostrils, indicating that there is an airway obstruction.

ongoing assessment The part of the assessment process in which problems are reevaluated and responses to treatment are assessed.

orientation The mental status of a patient; the patient's memory of person (his or her name), place (the current location), time (the current year, month, and approximate date), and event (what happened).

OPQRST The six pain questions: **O**nset, **P**rovoke, **Q**uality, **R**adiation, **S**everity, **T**ime and **T**reatment.

palpate Examine by touch.

paradoxical motion The motion of the chest wall that is detached in a flail chest; the motion is exactly the opposite of normal motion during breathing; that is, it is in during inhalation, out during exhalation.

penetrating trauma A mechanism of injury in which force occurs in a small point of contact between the skin and the object. The skin is broken and the potential for infection is high.

radiation A continuation of an area of pain or discomfort distal to the site of the origin of the pain.

rales Cracking, rattling breath sound that signals fluid in the air spaces of the lungs. Also called *crackles*.

responsiveness The way in which a patient responds to external stimuli, including verbal stimuli (sound), tactile stimuli (touch), and painful stimuli.

retractions Movements in which the skin pulls in around the ribs during inspiration.

rhonchi Coarse breath sounds heard in patients with chronic mucus in the airways.

SAMPLE history A key brief history of a patient's condition to determine **S**igns/**S**ymptoms, **A**llergies, **M**edications, **P**ertinent past history, **L**ast oral intake, and **E**vents leading to the illness/injury.

scene size-up The part of the assessment process in which a quick assessment of the scene and the surroundings is made to provide as much information as possible about the safety of the scene.

sclera The white portion of the eye; the tough outer coat of the eye that gives protection to the delicate, light-sensitive inner layer.

stridor A harsh, high-pitched inspiratory sound, such as the sound that is often heard in acute laryngeal (upper airway) obstruction.

subcutaneous emphysema The presence of air in soft tissues, causing a characteristic crackling sensation on palpation.

triage The process of establishing treatment and transportation priorities according to severity of injury and medical need.

two- to three-word dyspnea A condition in which a patient can speak only two to three words at a time without pausing to take a breath.

assessment in action

Moments after the fire department is called about a water flow alarm at the local high school, you and your partner are dispatched to the same address. Firefighters take only a few minutes to isolate the bathroom with the flaming wastebasket and put out the fire. They also find an 18-year-old man in one of the stalls, where he apparently sought refuge from the smoke and flames.

The firefighter who found him said that the patient was initially unresponsive and even now responds only by moaning when you pinch his arm. His pupils are dilated and barely reactive. His skin is warm, moist, and light gray-blue. He has a blood pressure of 104/66 mm Hg, a regular pulse of 130 beats/min, and respirations of 26/min.

1. Which of the following terms would best describe the patient's current level of consciousness?
   A. Alert and oriented
   B. Responsive to pain
   C. Semi-conscious
   D. Unresponsive
2. Which of the following characteristics of the patient's skin would suggest that the patient is not getting adequate oxygen?
   A. Pale
   B. Cyanotic
   C. Warm
   D. Moist
3. High-concentration supplemental oxygen would be best delivered to the patient by a:
   A. BVM device at 15 L/min.
   B. nasal cannula at 24 L/min.
   C. nonrebreathing mask at 15 L/min.
   D. pocket mask with connector tubing at 4 L/min.
4. Which of the following statements about assisted ventilations is true?
   A. An unresponsive patient who has adequate respirations must receive assisted ventilations with a BVM device.
   B. An unresponsive patient with respirations of 4/min should receive high-flow oxygen via nasal cannula.
   C. A patient who has inadequate respirations should receive highflow oxygen and receive assisted ventilations.
   D. A patient who is not breathing should receive 12 to 15 L of oxygen via a nonrebreathing mask.
5. Which of the following conditions is **NOT** considered to be a treatment priority in an adult patient?
   A. Unconscious and unresponsive to any form of stimuli
   B. Difficulty breathing and an altered level of consciousness
   C. Responsive only to pain and does not follow commands
   D. A systolic blood pressure of more than 120 mm Hg and leg pain

points to ponder

Objectives 3-2.5, 3-2.14, 3-2.19, 3-2.21

You and your partner arrive at the scene of a single-car rollover accident. You are first on the scene and find five victims. As you approach the vehicle, you stop at a patient who was thrown from the vehicle. This patient (patient A) has a weak pulse and irregular breathing and is missing about a third of her skull, with obvious brain damage. You continue to the car and find the driver (patient B) holding his arm, which is obviously fractured at midshaft humerus and is very painful. The next two patients are in the back seat. An approximately 10-year-old boy (passenger C) is unresponsive, and you can hear gurgling sounds when he breathes in. The other passenger in the back seat (passenger D) is an elderly woman with an open fracture of her femur, which is bleeding profusely. The last patient is an infant (passenger E), who has somehow become trapped under the front seat of the car. The infant is not making any noise and is not moving, but you are unable to access it quickly to check pulse or breathing. You complete your initial patient assessment and find no significant problems other than the ones listed above. Just you and your partner are present.

- In what order would you treat these patients, and why? Justify the order for each patient.

online outlook

During the initial assessment (ABC), life-threatening conditions are identified and their management is begun. You can learn more about the initial assessment by following the Trauma Assessment link at www.emtb.com.

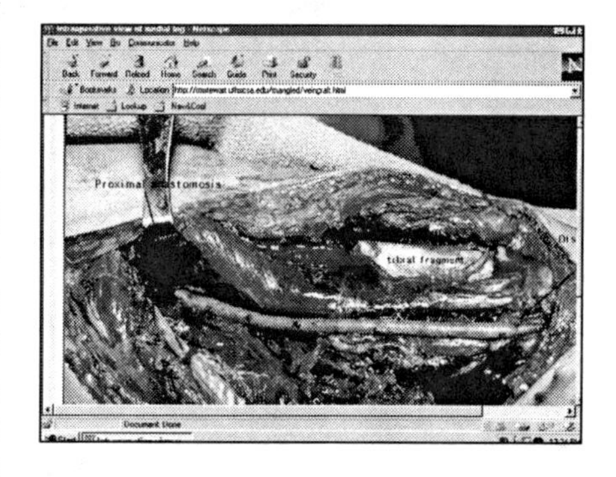

Baseline Vital Signs and SAMPLE History

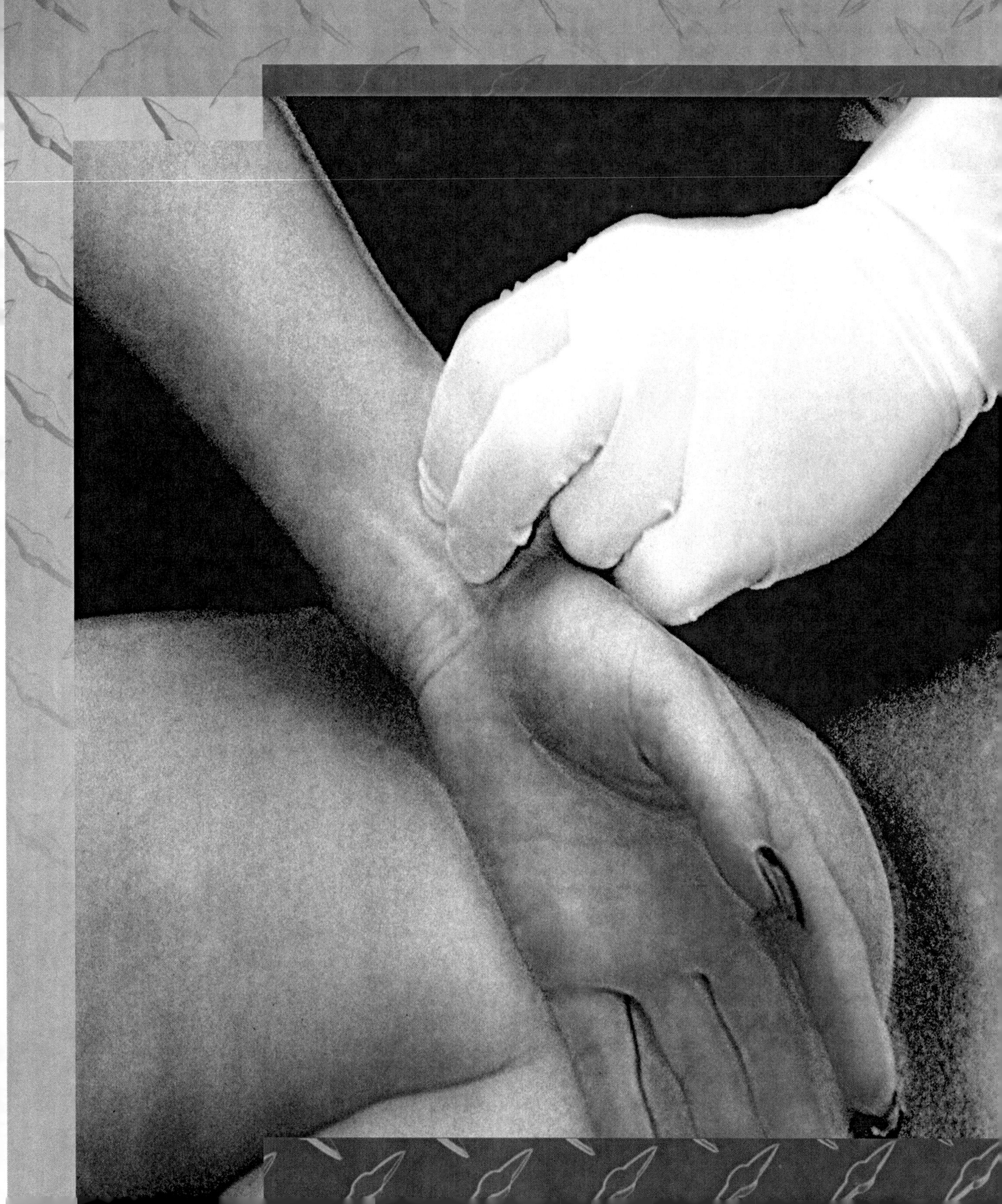

chapter 2

objectives

Cognitive

1. Identify the components of vital signs.
2. Describe the methods to obtain a breathing rate.
3. Identify the attributes that should be obtained when assessing breathing.
4. Differentiate between shallow, labored, and noisy breathing.
5. Describe the methods to obtain a pulse rate.
6. Identify the information obtained when assessing a patient's pulse.
7. Differentiate between a strong, weak, regular, and irregular pulse.
8. Describe the methods to assess the skin color, temperature, condition (capillary refill in infants and children).
9. Identify the normal and abnormal skin colors.
10. Differentiate between pale, blue, red, and yellow skin color.
11. Identify the normal and abnormal skin temperature.
12. Differentiate between hot, cool, and cold skin temperature.
13. Identify normal and abnormal skin conditions.
14. Identify normal and abnormal capillary refill in infants and children.
15. Describe the methods to assess the pupils.
16. Identify normal and abnormal pupil size.
17. Differentiate between dilated (big) and constricted (small) pupil size.
18. Differentiate between reactive and nonreactive pupils and equal and unequal pupils.
19. Describe the methods to assess blood pressure.
20. Define systolic pressure.
21. Define diastolic pressure.
22. Explain the difference between auscultation and palpation for obtaining a blood pressure.
23. Identify the components of the SAMPLE history.
24. Differentiate between a sign and a symptom.
25. State the importance of accurately reporting and recording the baseline vital signs.
26. Discuss the need to search for additional medical identification.

Affective

27. Explain the value of performing the baseline vital signs.
28. Recognize and respond to the feelings patients experience during assessment.
29. Defend the need for obtaining and recording an accurate set of vital signs.
30. Explain the rationale of recording additional sets of vital signs.
31. Explain the importance of obtaining a SAMPLE history.

Psychomotor

32. Demonstrate the skills involved in assessment of breathing.
33. Demonstrate the skills associated with obtaining a pulse.
34. Demonstrate the skills associated with assessing the skin color, temperature, condition, and capillary refill in infants and children.
35. Demonstrate the skills associated with assessing the pupils.
36. Demonstrate the skills associated with obtaining blood pressure.
37. Demonstrate the skills that should be used to obtain information from the patient, family, or bystanders at the scene.

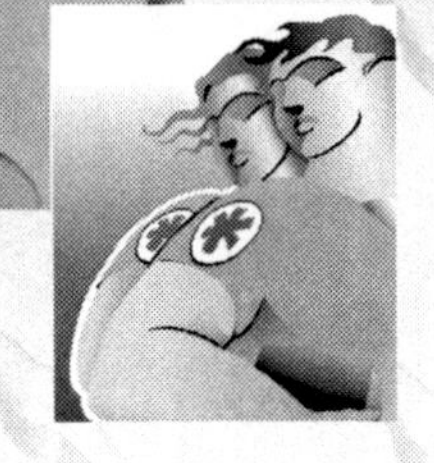

you are the cfr/emt

Squad 12, report to Sunnydale Care Facility for a special assignment. You have been assigned to Blood Pressure Day. Your partner groans, "Why are these folks so concerned about their weekly blood pressure check?" "It's good preventive medicine. You have to know the normal pressure to identify the abnormal." Your philosophical answer leaves your partner thinking quietly as you get into your unit to drive to Sunnydale.

This chapter describes the importance of obtaining and evaluating baseline vital signs and the SAMPLE history. It will also help you to answer the following questions:

1. Should vital signs be absolutely accurate, or are approximate readings sufficient?
2. When should you first obtain vital signs? After that, how often should you obtain them?

Baseline Vital Signs and SAMPLE History

As an EMT-B, you must perform a quick but thorough assessment to identify a patient's needs and to provide proper emergency medical care. Patient assessment includes many steps and is the most complex skill that you will learn in the EMT-B course. To make the task easier, it is helpful to identify and discuss the key components and skills of patient assessment before you learn the entire process.

As you begin your assessment, you must gather and record some key information about the patient. You will also need to obtain and evaluate the patient's vital signs. The injuries, illnesses, or symptoms that lead to the call to 9-1-1 and the history of what occurred before and since the call was made are key pieces of information that you will have to obtain by asking a series of questions. You must also learn about the patient's past medical history and overall health.

This chapter begins by defining the chief complaint and signs and symptoms. It then explains what key information about the patient you need to obtain at the start of the assessment and why you need it. It also describes each of the vital signs and provides a step-by-step explanation of how to obtain each. Both normal and abnormal vital signs are discussed. The chapter ends with a description of the SAMPLE history.

Gathering Key Patient Information

During the assessment, you will be using your eyes, ears, nose, hands, and a few basic medical instruments to obtain information about your patient. You will need to know which questions to ask and how to ask them (Figure 5-1). By using your deductive powers, you will be able to interpret the meaning and implications of your findings and the information that you have gathered. When assessing the patient, you will have to look, listen, feel, and think. Your scene size-up or the information that is given to you by a first responder or relative when you arrive at the scene should make it immediately apparent whether you were called to the scene because of an accident with injuries or an acute medical problem.

As you begin the physical examination, you should ask another EMT-B, if available, to obtain the patient's full name, address, age, gender, and race and to record

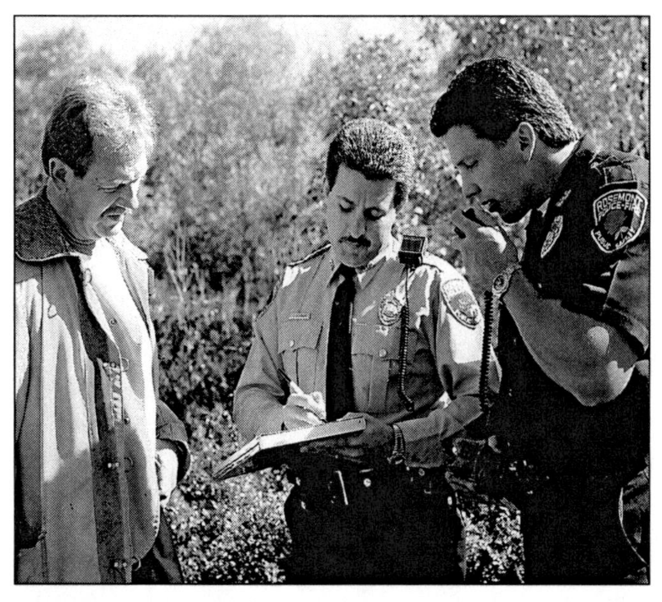

FIGURE 5-1 You must know how to gather information about the scene and the patient by using your senses and by asking relevant questions.

them on the run report. This information may be important if the patient later loses consciousness or becomes disoriented, and it helps the hospital staff to retrieve past medical records. However, *collection of this information is not a priority.* You must not lose sight of the initial assessment and its purpose.

You will also need some of this information in the field. You will need to know the patient's name so that you can properly address the patient. Unless an adult patient is a close friend or relative of yours, you should address him or her as "Mr.," "Ms.," "Miss," or "Mrs.," followed by the patient's last name. You may ask the patient how he or she wishes to be called. Often, relatives or staff members of a nursing home or other extended care facility address elderly patients by their first names. You should not use such a familiar mode of address. If the patient's name is difficult to pronounce, you can simply say "Sir" or "Ma'am" instead, to convey a similar respectful and professional manner.

You should try to address children by their first name, especially the name they are customarily called, such as "Johnny," "Betty," or "Joey." Even infants and toddlers who do not yet respond verbally can recognize their name and may be less anxious when it is used.

If an unaccompanied patient is disoriented or unconscious, you should look in his or her wallet or purse for a driver's license or other piece of identification that will tell you the patient's name. At the same time, you should check for any hospital identification or medical alert card. *Always* look for patient identification in the presence of another EMT or law enforcement officer at the scene.

Age and gender are also important considerations in assessing a patient. Some conditions and illnesses are found predominantly in younger patients; others are commonly found only in older patients. Some conditions are prevalent in a certain age group in adult men but in a different age group in women. Some are more prevalent in one gender, and some are limited exclusively to either male or female patients. In addition, the normal range of some of the vital signs will be different for different age groups of children, adults, and elderly patients.

Chief Complaint/ Mechanism of Injury

The reason that a patient or others call 9-1-1 is vital information. This reason is called the patient's chief complaint. In the most literal definition, chief complaints are the major signs and symptoms that the patient reports when asked, "What seems to be the matter?" or "What's wrong?" A patient who responds "My chest hurts" is stating the chief complaint. What you see must also be considered in determining the chief complaint. If the patient's response demonstrates that he or she is having significant difficulty breathing, "difficulty breathing" should be included in the chief complaint as if the patient had reported it verbally. In some protocols, a chief complaint also includes any significant gross, apparent injuries.

The problems or feelings the patients reports to you, such as " I feel dizzy," "My leg hurts," or "Ow, that hurts a lot!" are called symptoms. These cannot be felt or observed by others. The severity of a symptom is subjective because it is based on the patient's interpretation and tolerance. Signs are conditions that can be seen, heard, felt, smelled, or measured by you or others. Wounds, external bleeding, marked deformities, respirations, and pulse are all signs (Figure 5-2).

Signs and symptoms that occurred before you arrived, such as dizziness that resulted in a loss of consciousness,

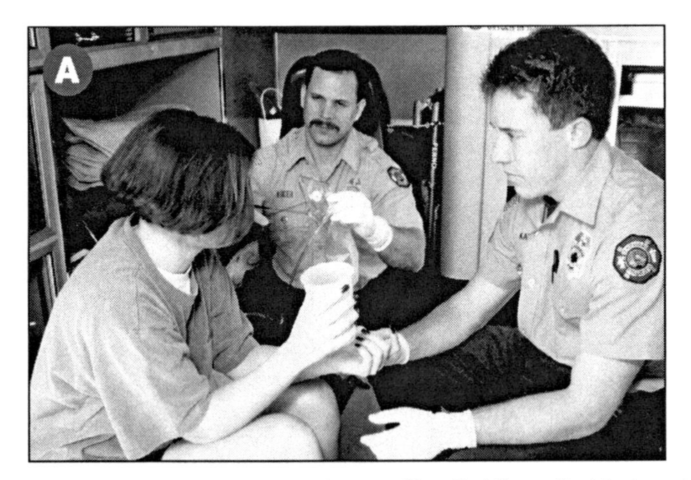

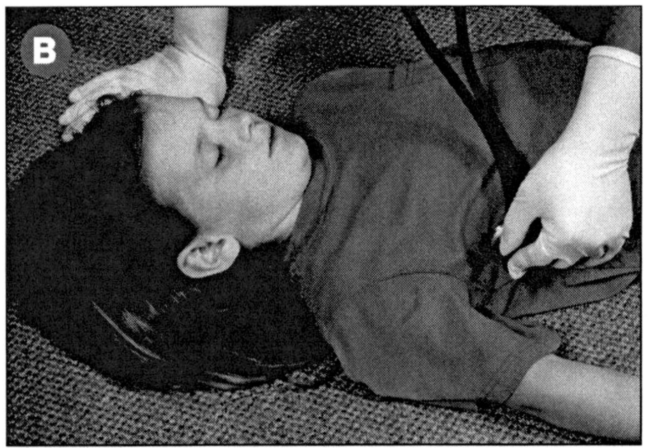

FIGURE 5-2 A: A symptom is a condition that the patient feels and tells you about. **B:** A sign is condition that you can observe about the patient.

may be reported by the patient or others at the scene. Because signs and symptoms are essential to understanding the sequence of events and may include signs that are no longer present, they are important parts of the patient history. You should always report how and/or when the signs and symptoms began. This information is important because the reason that signs and symptoms develop often differs, depending on the situation.

Baseline Vital Signs

The initial assessment is a rapid evaluation of the patient's general condition to identify any potentially life-threatening conditions. The brain and other vital organs require constant oxygen. Significant problems with breathing or circulation must be considered potentially life-threatening conditions. A critical problem or deficit in any of the body's other vital systems or functions will progressively affect and be reflected by changes in the respiratory, circulatory, and central nervous systems. Therefore, the status of these three systems serves as your guideline for evaluating and measuring the patient's general condition.

Vital signs are the key signs that are used to evaluate the patient's initial general condition. The first set of vital signs that you obtain is called the *baseline vital signs*. By periodically reassessing the vital signs and comparing the findings with the baseline set, you will be able to identify any significant trends in the patient's condition, particularly whether the patient's condition is becoming worse (Figure 5-3).

Because key indicators include a quantitative (numeric) objective measurement, you will always include the patient's respirations, pulse, and blood pressure when taking and evaluating the vital signs. Other key indications of the patient's respiratory, cardiovascular, and central nervous system status include evaluation of the following:

- Skin temperature and condition in adults
- Capillary refill in children
- Pupillary reaction
- Level of consciousness

Respirations

A patient who is breathing independently is said to have spontaneous respirations or spontaneous ventilations. Each complete breath includes two distinct phases: inspiration and expiration. During inspiration (inhalation), the chest rises up and out, drawing oxygenated air into the alveoli in the lungs. During expiration (exhalation), the chest returns to its original position, releasing air with an increased carbon dioxide level out of the lungs. Inhalation and exhalation times occur in a 1:3 ratio; the active inhalation phase lasts one third the amount of time of the passive exhalation phase.

Breathing is a continuous process in which each breath regularly follows the last with no notable interruption. Breathing is normally a spontaneous automatic process that occurs without conscious thought, visible effort, marked sounds, or pain. You will assess breathing by watching the patient's chest rise and fall, feeling for air through the mouth and nose during exhalation, and listening to breath sounds with a stethoscope over each lung. Chest rise and breath sounds should be equal on both sides of the chest. A conscious patient who is speaking has spontaneous respirations.

When assessing respirations, you must determine the rate, depth, and quality (character) of the patient's breathing.

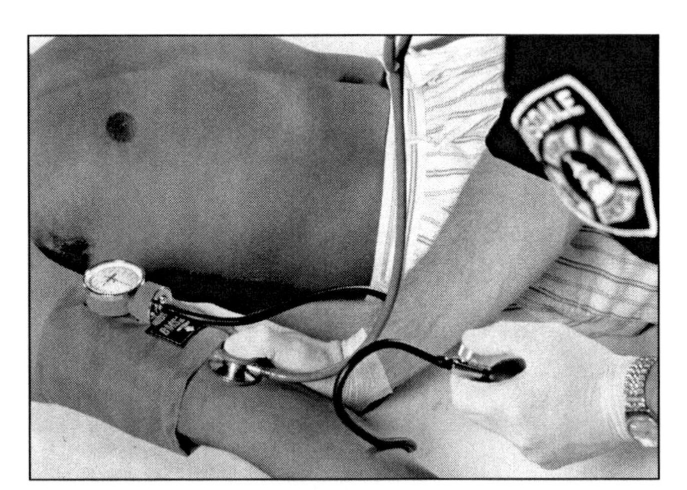

FIGURE 5-3 Baseline vital signs are key signs that are used to evaluate the patient's initial condition.

timing the respirations or pulse rate

When timing a patient's respirations or pulse rate, count the number of breaths or beats in a 30-second period and then multiply by 2. This method produces a significantly more reliable figure than you would get if you counted for only 15 seconds and multiplied by 4. With either method, the result will always be an even number.

You might find it easier to count if you use an analog watch with a sweep second hand or a digital watch with a stopwatch function.

> When assessing respirations, you must determine the rate, depth, and quality (character) of the patient's breathing.

Rate. Respirations are determined by counting the number of breaths in a 30-second period and multiplying by 2. The result equals the number of breaths per minute. For accuracy, you should count each breath at the same point in its cycle. This is most easily done by counting each peak chest rise. Although you can see peak chest rise, it is easier to place your hand on the patient's chest and feel it. However, be aware that a conscious patient who knows that you are evaluating his or her breathing will often override the automatic rate and depth by breathing more slowly and deeply. To prevent this from happening, you should check respirations in a conscious, alert patient without making the patient aware of what you are evaluating. This can be easily done by first taking a radial pulse and then, without releasing the wrist or otherwise suggesting a change, counting the chest rise that you see or feel as the patient's forearm rises and falls with the movement of the chest (Figure 5-4). If the patient coughs, yawns, sighs, or talks during the 30-second period, you should wait a few seconds and start again. Table 5-1 shows the normal range of respiratory rates of patients who are at rest.

Normal respirations can vary greatly. In a well-conditioned athlete, normal respirations may be as low as 6 to 8 breaths/min.

Quality. You can determine the quality or character of respirations as you are counting. Table 5-2 shows the four ways in which the quality or character can be described.

Rhythm. While counting the patient's respirations, you should also note the rhythm. If the time from one peak chest rise to the next is fairly consistent, respirations are considered regular. If respirations vary or change frequently, they are considered irregular. When you document the vital signs, be sure to note whether the patient's respirations were regular or irregular.

Depth. The amount of air that the patient is exchanging depends on both the rate and the tidal volume, the amount of air that is exchanged with each breath. The depth of the breath determines whether the tidal volume is normal, less than normal, or more than normal. Respirations are described as shallow when the movement of the chest wall and air that you feel exhaled with each breath is less than normal. Deep respirations occur

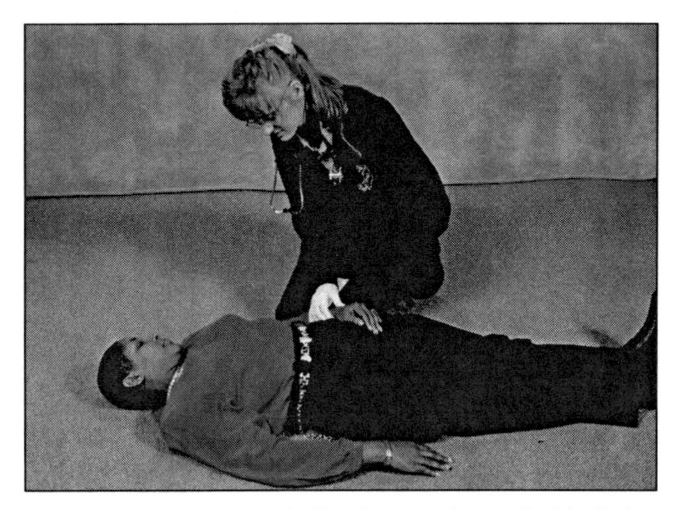

FIGURE 5-4 Assess respirations in a conscious patient by first taking a radial pulse and then, without releasing the patient's wrist, counting the chest rise and fall for 30 seconds.

TABLE 5-1 Normal Ranges for Respirations

Age	Range
Adults	12 to 20 breaths/min
Children	15 to 30 breaths/min
Infants	25 to 50 breaths/min

TABLE 5-2 Characteristics of Respirations

Normal	Breathing is neither shallow nor deep Average chest wall motion No use of accessory muscles
Shallow	Slight chest or abdominal wall motion
Labored	Increased breathing effort Grunting, stridor Use of accessory muscles Possible gasping Nasal flaring, supraclavicular and intercostal retractions in infants and children
Noisy	Increase in sound of breathing, including snoring, wheezing, gurgling, and crowing

when chest movement and exhaled air are significantly greater than normal. You should document when the patient's respirations are shallow or deep; however, you do not have to record a normal depth of breathing.

caring for kids

Chest rise in a small child is less marked than that in an adult. However, a small child's abdomen moves more with each breath than an adult's does. Place your hands on the outer margin of the lower anterior chest to feel the chest wall and abdominal movement, and determine whether the depth is normal, shallow, or deep. In a patient of any age, if it is difficult to gauge the depth of breathing from the chest movement, note instead the amount of air that you feel is exhaled with each breath.

Effort. Normally, breathing is an effortless process that does not affect a patient's speech, posture, or positioning. Speech is a good indicator of whether a conscious patient is having difficulty breathing. A patient who can speak smoothly without unusual extra pauses is breathing normally. However, a patient who can speak only one word at a time or must stop every two to three words to catch his or her breath is having significant difficulty breathing. Patients who are having marked difficulty breathing will instinctively assume a posture in which it is easier for them to breathe. This is called the sniffing position or tripod position. In this position, a patient sits unusually upright with the head and chin thrust slightly forward and is having sufficient difficulty breathing that a significant marked conscious effort is required (Figure 5-5) .

Breathing that becomes progressively more difficult requires progressively more effort. When you can see that effort, the patient's breathing is described as labored breathing.

Initially, labored breathing is characterized by the patient's position, concentration on breathing, and the increased effort and depth of each breath. As breathing becomes progressively more labored, accessory muscles in the face and neck are used, and the patient may make some grunting sounds with each breath. In infants and small children, nasal flaring and *supraclavicular* and *intercostal retractions* (indentation above the clavicles and in the spaces between the ribs) are commonly associated with labored breathing. Sometimes, the patient may be gasping.

Infants and small children will continue to have labored breathing for a sustained period, will then often become exhausted, and finally will no longer have the strength to maintain the necessary energy to breathe. These patients will then appear to breathe normally again, even though the amount of ventilation is insufficient; however, their respirations will progressively decline until respiratory arrest develops. In infants and small children, cardiac arrest is generally caused by respiratory arrest.

Noisy breathing. Normal breathing is silent or, in a very quiet environment, accompanied only by the sounds of air movement at the mouth and nose. Through a stethoscope, normal breath sounds include only the sound of air movement through the bronchi accompanied by a soft, low-pitched murmur. Breathing accompanied by other sounds indicates a significant respiratory problem. When the airway is partially obstructed by a foreign body, fluid, or swelling, you may hear stridor, a harsh, high-pitched, crowing sound. If you can hear bubbling or gurgling, the patient probably has fluid in the airway. With a complete airway obstruction, the patient will not be able to pass any air and will no longer be able to cough or talk. You may hear other sounds, including wheezes, snoring, gur-

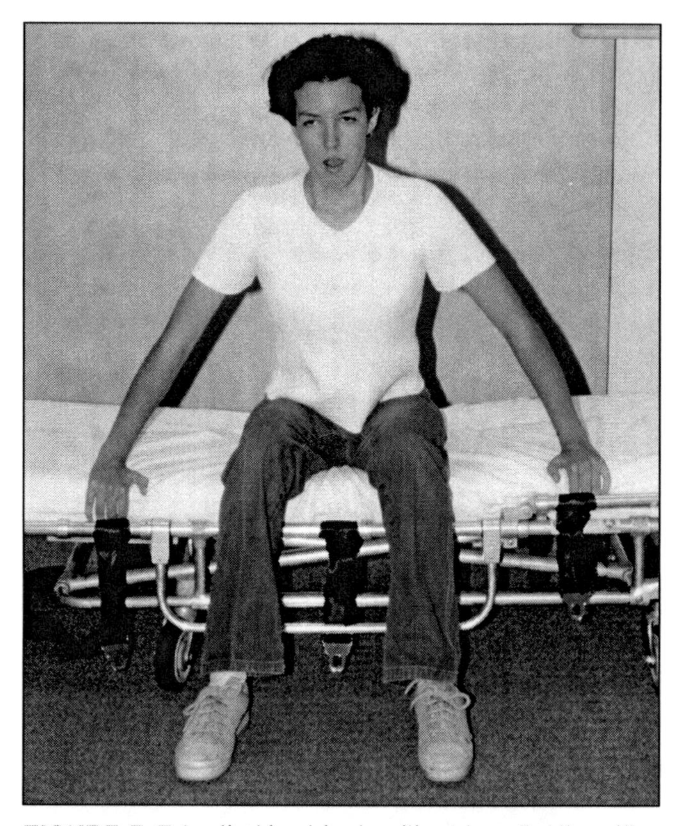

FIGURE 5-5 A patient in a tripod position (also called the sniffing position) will sit unusually upright with the head and chin thrust forward slightly.

gling, or bubbling. The presence of any of these indicates that a serious respiratory problem exists.

A patient who coughs up thick, yellowish or greenish *sputum* (matter from the lungs) most likely has an advanced respiratory infection. A patient with a chest injury may cough up blood or a frothy whitish or pinkish foamlike sputum. A patient with congestive heart failure may also cough up a frothy sputum. The presence of either substance, regardless of its cause, indicates that an urgent, potentially critical cardiovascular and respiratory problem exists. The patient's condition may deteriorate rapidly to a point at which the patient can no longer breathe.

Pulse

With each heartbeat, the ventricles contract, forcefully ejecting blood from the heart and propelling it into the arteries. The pulse is the pressure wave that occurs as each heartbeat causes a surge in the blood circulating through the arteries. The pulse is most easily felt at a pulse point where a major artery lies near the surface and can be pressed gently against a bone or solid organ. To *palpate* (feel) the pulse, hold together your index and long fingers and place their tips over a pulse point, pressing gently against the artery until you feel intermittent pulsations. Sometimes, you may have to slide your fingertips a little to each side and press again until you feel a pulse. When palpating a pulse, do not allow your thumb to touch the patient. If you do so, you may mistake the strong pulsing circulation in your thumb for the patient's pulse.

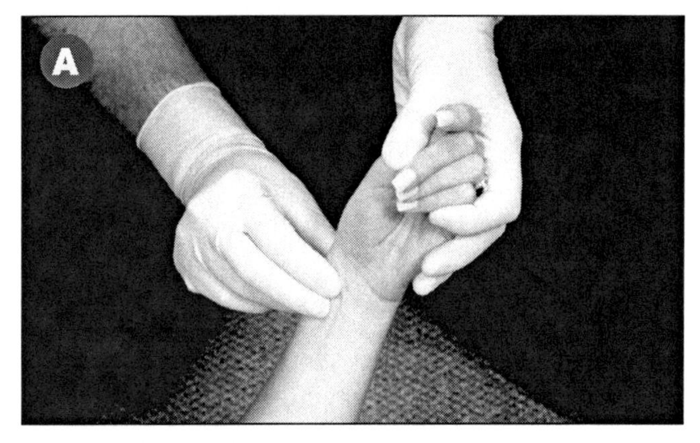

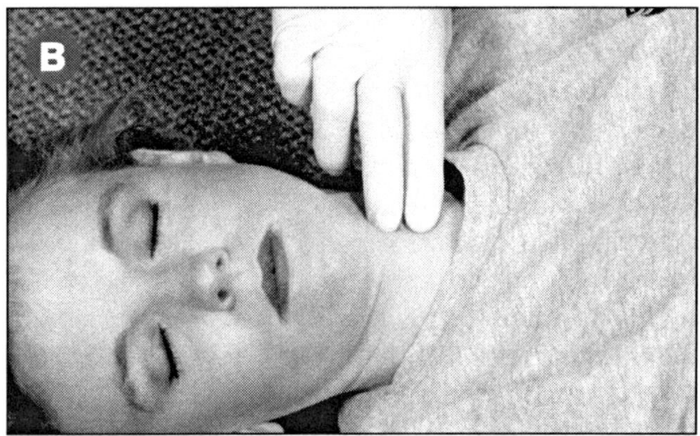

FIGURE 5-6 A: To palpate the radial pulse, place the tips of your first two fingers over the radial artery, pressing gently until you feel intermittent pulsations. **B:** To palpate the carotid pulse, place the tips of your first two fingers over the carotid artery, pressing gently until you feel intermittent pulsations.

In responsive patients who are older than age 1 year, you should palpate the radial pulse at the wrist (Figure 5-6). In unresponsive patients older than age 1 year, you should palpate the carotid pulse in the neck, which is easier to locate. When palpating the carotid pulse, you should place the fingertips of your index and long fingers along the carotid artery. Use caution when palpating the carotid pulse in a responsive patient, especially an elderly patient. Only gentle pressure on one side of the neck should be used. Never press on the carotid arteries on both sides of the neck at the same time. Doing so can cut off circulation to the brain.

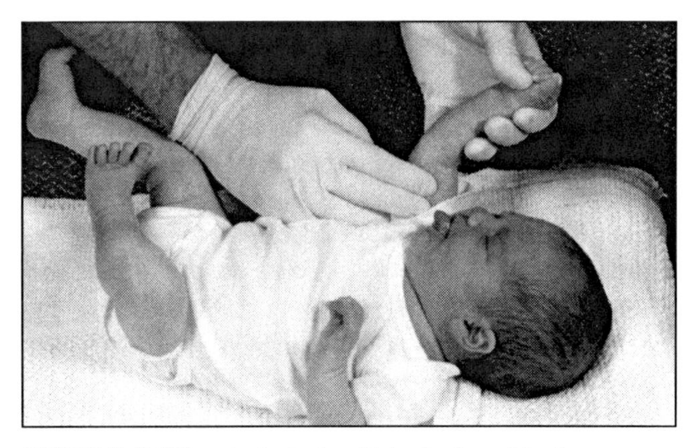

FIGURE 5-7 To palpate the brachial pulse in an infant, press firmly along the brachial artery at the underside of the upper arm.

In infants, both the radial and carotid pulses are difficult to locate. Because of the infant's soft, immature trachea, palpating the carotid pulse is not recommended. Palpate the brachial pulse, located at the underside of the upper arm, in children younger than age 1 year (Figure 5-7). With the infant lying supine, you can access the brachial pulse by elevating the arm over the infant's head. Because most infants have chubby arms, you need to press your adjacent fingertips firmly along the brachial artery, which lies parallel to the long axis of the upper arm, to be able to palpate the pulse.

Your first consideration when taking a pulse is to determine whether the patient has a palpable pulse or is pulseless. When taking the pulse, you should assess and report its rate, strength, and regularity.

TABLE 5-3 Normal Ranges for Pulse Rate

Age	Range
Adults	60 to 100 beats/min
Children	80 to 100 beats/min
Toddlers	100 to 120 beats/min
Newborns	120 to 140 beats/min

Rate. To obtain the pulse rate in most patients, you should count the number of pulses felt in a 30-second period and then multiply by 2. A pulse that is weak and difficult to palpate, irregular, or extremely slow should be palpated and counted for a full minute. A pulse rate is counted as beats per minute; however, in reporting the pulse rate, it is not necessary to state or write "beats per minute" after the number.

The pulse rate in most adults (at rest) averages around 72 beats/min. However, pulse rate can vary significantly from person to person. In the well-conditioned athlete or in individuals taking heart medications such as beta-blockers, the pulse rate may be considerably lower. A pulse rate between 60 and 100 beats/min is considered normal in adults. The average pulse rate in children is generally higher. Table 5-3 shows the normal ranges of pulse rates.

In assessing the pulse rate in an adult patient, a rate that is greater than 100 beats/min is described as tachycardia, and a rate of less than 60 beats/min is described as bradycardia.

Strength. You should always report the pulse's strength and regularity whenever reporting or recording the pulse. The pulse is generally palpated at the radial or carotid arteries in adults and at the brachial artery in infants, because it is normally strong and easily palpable at these locations. Therefore, if the pulse feels of normal strength, you should describe it as being strong. You should describe a stronger than normal pulse as "bounding" and a pulse that is weak and difficult to feel as "weak" or "thready." With a little experience, you will be able to make the necessary distinctions easily.

Regularity. When assessing the quality of the pulse, you must also determine whether it is regular or irregular. When the interval between each ventricular contraction of the heart is short, the pulse is rapid. When the interval is longer, the pulse is slower. No matter what the rate, the interval between each contraction should be the same, and the pulse that results should occur at a constant, regular rhythm. You should note and document this rhythm as regular.

The rhythm is considered irregular if the heart periodically has a premature or late beat or if a pulse beat is missed. Some individuals have a chronically irregular pulse; however, if an irregular pulse is found in a patient with signs and symptoms that suggest a cardiovascular problem, the patient likely needs advanced cardiac assessment and life support. Therefore, depending on your protocols, you should call for ALS backup, arrange for an intercept, or initiate prompt transport to definitive care.

The Skin

The condition of the patient's skin can tell you a lot about the patient's peripheral circulation and perfusion, blood oxygen levels, and body temperature. When assessing the skin, you should evaluate its color, temperature, and moisture.

Color. Assessing the skin helps you to determine the adequacy of perfusion after trauma. Perfusion is the circulation of blood within an organ or tissue. Adequate perfusion meets the cells' current needs; inadequate perfusion will cause cells and tissues to die.

Many blood vessels lie near the surface of the skin. The skin's color is determined by the blood circulating through these vessels and the amount and type of pigment that is present in the skin. Blood is red when it is properly saturated with oxygen. As a result, skin in lightly pigmented individuals is pinkish. The pigmentation in most individuals will not hide changes in the skin's underlying color, regardless of the individual's race. In patients with deeply pigmented skin, changes in color may be apparent only in certain areas, such as the fingernail beds, the mucous membranes in the mouth, the lips, the underside of the arm and palm (which are usually less pigmented), and the conjunctiva of the eyes. In addition, the palms of the hands and soles of the feet should be assessed in infants and children.

Poor peripheral circulation will cause the skin to appear pale, white, ashen or gray, possibly with a waxy translucent appearance like a white candle. Abnormally cold or frozen skin may also appear this way. When the blood is not properly saturated with oxygen, it appears bluish. Therefore, in a patient with insufficient air exchange and low levels of oxygen in the blood, the blood and vessels become bluish, and the lips, mucous membranes, nail beds, and skin over the blood vessels appear blue or gray. This condition is called cyanosis (Figure 5-8).

High blood pressure will cause the skin to be abnormally flushed and red. In some patients with extremely high blood pressure, all the visible blood vessels will be so full that the skin will appear to be a dark reddish-

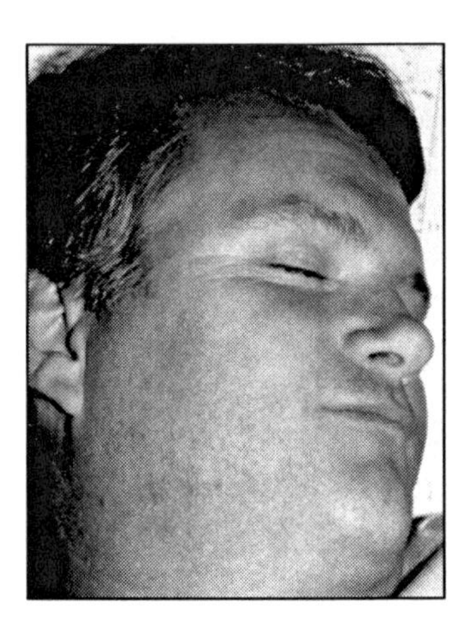

FIGURE 5-8 Cyanosis occurs when the patient has low levels of oxygen in the blood.

purple. A patient with carbon monoxide poisoning or a significant fever, heatstroke, sunburn, mild thermal burns, or other conditions in which the body is unable to properly dissipate heat will also appear to have red skin.

Changes in skin color may also result from chronic illness. Liver disease or dysfunction may cause jaundice, resulting in the patient's skin and sclera turning yellow.

Temperature. Normally, the skin is warm to the touch. When the patient has a significant fever, sunburn, or hyperthermia, the skin feels hot to the touch. The skin will feel cool when the patient is in early shock, has exercised and is sweating profusely, or has heat exhaustion. The skin will feel cold when the patient is in profound shock, has hypothermia, or has frostbite.

Body temperature is normally measured with a thermometer in the hospital. However, in the field, feeling the patient's forehead with the back of your hand is usually adequate to determine whether the patient's temperature is elevated or depressed (Figure 5-9).

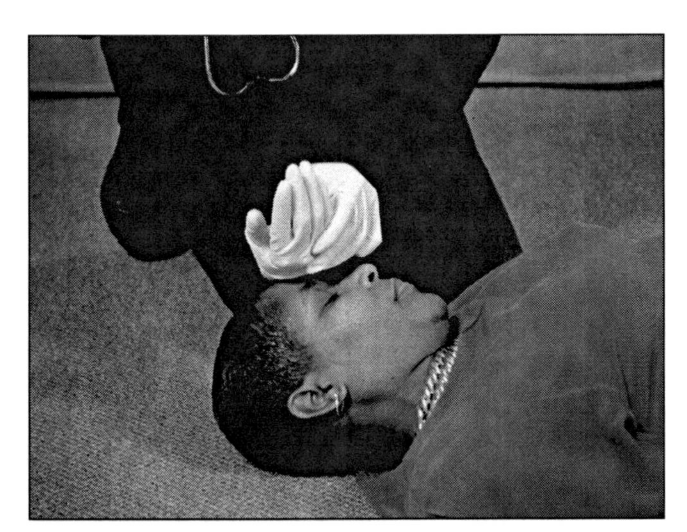

FIGURE 5-9 Assess skin temperature by feeling the patient's forehead with the back of your hand.

Moisture. Dry skin is normal. Skin that is wet, moist (often called diaphoretic), or excessively dry and hot suggests a problem. In the early stages of shock, the skin will become slightly moist. Skin that is only slightly moist but not covered excessively with sweat is described as clammy, damp, or moist. When the skin is bathed in sweat, such as after strenuous exercise or when the patient is in the late stages of shock, the skin is described as wet.

Because the skin's color, temperature, and moisture are often related signs, you should consider them together. When recording or reporting your assessment of the skin, you should first describe the color, then the temperature, and last, whether the skin is dry, moist, or wet. For example, you could say or write, "Skin: pale, cool, and clammy."

Capillary Refill

Capillary refill is a test that evaluates the ability of the circulatory system to restore blood to the capillary system. When evaluated in an uninjured limb, capillary refill reflects the patient's perfusion. Capillary refill time is often affected by the patient's body temperature, position, and medications. To test capillary refill, place your thumb on the patient's fingernail with your fingers on the underside of the patient's finger, and gently compress (Figure 5-10). The blood will be forced from the

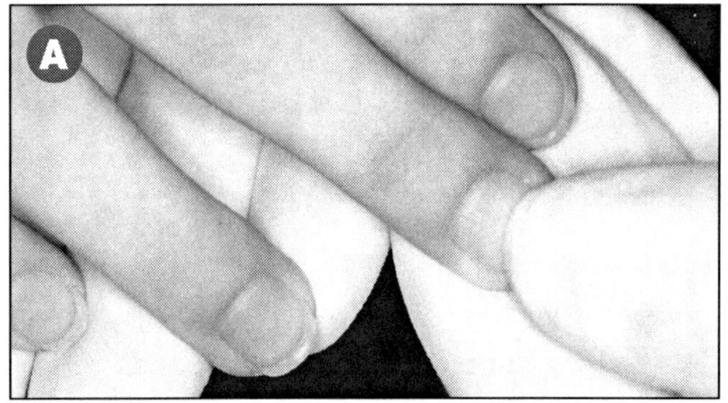

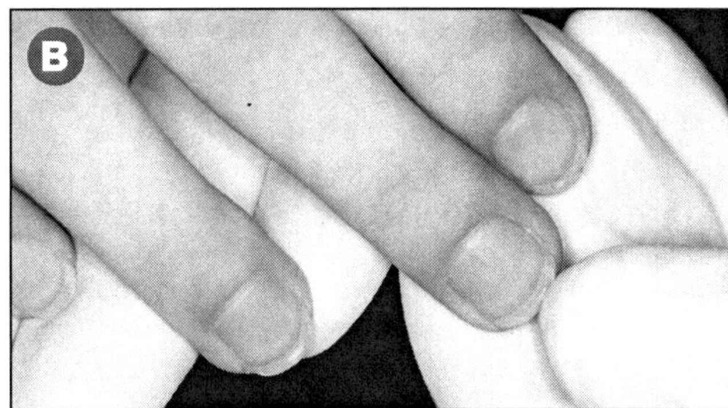

FIGURE 5-10 **A:** To test capillary refill, gently compress the fingertip until it blanches. **B:** Release the fingertip, and count until it returns to its normal pink color.

capillaries in the nail bed. When you remove the pressure applied against the tip of the patient's finger, the nail bed will remain blanched and white for a brief period. As the underlying capillaries refill with blood, the nail bed will be restored to its normal deep pink color. Capillary refill should be both prompt and pink. With adequate perfusion, the color in the nail bed should be restored to its normal pink within 2 seconds, or about the time it takes to say "capillary refill" at a normal rate of speech. You should report and document the capillary refill as normal. You should suspect poor peripheral circulation when capillary refill takes more than 2 seconds or the nail bed remains blanched. In this instance, you should report and document the capillary refill as delayed.

A bluish color may indicate that the capillaries are refilling with blood drawn from the veins rather than with fresh, oxygenated blood from the arteries, making the test invalid. You should also consider the capillary refill test invalid if the patient is in or has been exposed to a cold environment or if the patient is elderly. In both situations, delayed capillary refill is normal.

To assess capillary refill in infants and children younger than age 6 years, press on the skin or nail bed, and determine how long it takes for the pink color to return. As with adults, normal capillary refill takes less than 2 seconds.

Blood Pressure

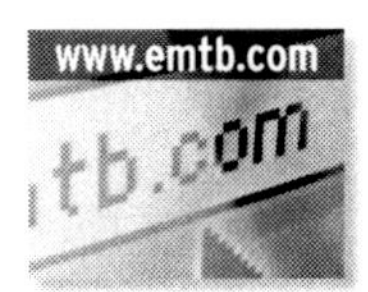

Adequate blood pressure is necessary to maintain proper circulation and perfusion of the vital organ cells. Blood pressure (BP) is the pressure of circulating blood against the walls of the arteries. A decrease in the blood pressure may indicate one of the following:

- Loss of blood or its fluid components
- Loss of vascular tone and sufficient arterial constriction to maintain the necessary pressure even without any actual fluid or blood loss
- A cardiac pumping problem

When any of these conditions occurs and results in a small drop in circulation, the body's compensatory mechanisms are activated, the heart and pulse rates increase, and the arteries constrict. Normal blood pressure is maintained, and by decreasing the blood flow to the skin and extremities, available blood volume is temporarily redirected to the vital organs so that they remain adequately perfused. However, as shock progresses, and the body's defense mechanisms can no longer keep up, the blood pressure will fall. *Decreased blood pressure is a late sign of shock and indicates that the critical decompensated phase has begun.* Any patient with a markedly low blood pressure has inadequate pressure to maintain proper perfusion of all the vital organs and needs to have his or her blood pressure and perfusion restored immediately to a normal level.

When the blood pressure becomes elevated, the body's defenses act to reduce it. Some individuals have chronically high blood pressure from progressive narrowing of the arteries that occurs with age, and during an acute episode, their blood pressure may increase to even higher levels. Head injury or a number of other conditions may also cause blood pressure to rise to very high levels. Abnormally high blood pressure may result in a rupture or other critical damage in the arterial system.

You should measure blood pressure in all patients older than age 3 years. In addition to baseline vital signs, you should note a sick appearance, respiratory distress, or unresponsiveness when evaluating infants and children younger than age 3 years.

Blood pressure contains two key separate components: diastolic pressure and systolic pressure. Diastolic pressure is the residual pressure that remains in the arteries during the relaxing phase (diastole) of the heart's cycle, when the left ventricle is at rest. Systolic pressure is the increased pressure that is caused along the artery with each contraction (systole) of the ventricle and the pulse wave that it produces. Systolic pressure represents the maximum pressure to which the arteries are subjected, and the diastolic pressure represents the minimum amount of pressure that is always present in the arteries.

Early blood pressure gauges contained a column of mercury and a linear scale that was graduated in millimeters. Even though different gauges are used today, the blood pressure is still measured in millimeters of mercury (mm Hg). Blood pressure is reported as a fraction in the form systolic pressure over diastolic pressure. Therefore, if the patient's systolic pressure is 120 and the diastolic pressure is 78, you would record it as "BP 120/78 mm Hg." You would report the patient's blood pressure verbally as "BP is 120 over 78."

Blood pressure contains two key separate components: diastolic pressure and systolic pressure.

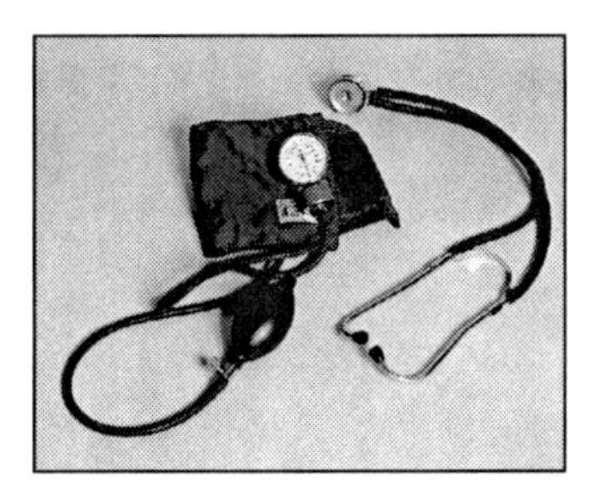

FIGURE 5-11
A blood pressure cuff.

Equipment for measuring blood pressure. You will use a *sphygmomanometer* (blood pressure cuff) to apply pressure against the artery when measuring the blood pressure. The sphygmomanometer contains the following components (Figure 5-11):

- A wide outer cuff designed to be fastened snugly around the entire arm or leg
- An inflatable wide bladder sewn into a portion of the cuff
- A ball-pump with a one-way valve that allows air to enter and a turn-valve that can be closed or, when opened, will allow air to be released at a controlled speed from the cuff
- A pressure gauge calibrated in millimeters of mercury, which indicates the pressure that exists in the cuff that is being applied against the underlying artery

Make sure that you carry at least three sizes of blood pressure cuffs: normal, extra-large, and pediatric (Figure 5-12). The normal size cuff is designed to adjust properly around the upper arm of most adults. Use an extra-large cuff with patients who are obese or have exceptionally well-developed arm muscles or to take the blood pressure of the thigh in patients who have injuries in both arms. Use a narrow, small pediatric cuff with children and exceptionally small adults.

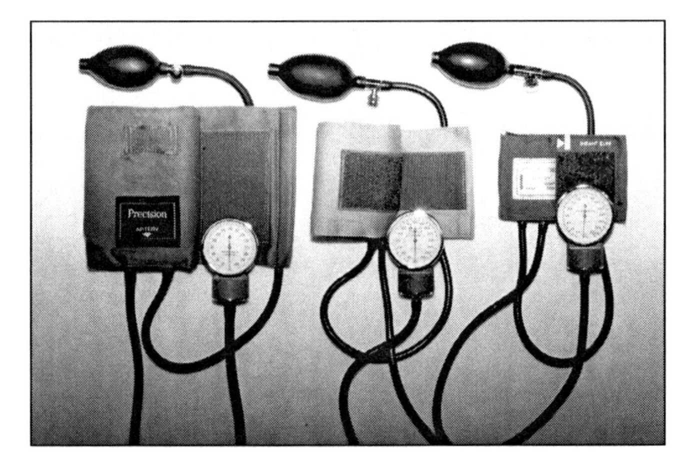

FIGURE 5-12 The three sizes of blood pressure cuffs: extra-large, normal, and pediatric.

You must be sure to select the appropriately sized cuff. A cuff that is too small may result in falsely high readings; a cuff that is too large may result in falsely low readings.

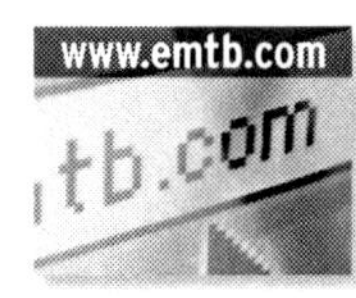

Auscultation. Auscultation is the method of listening to sounds within organs with a stethoscope. You will usually measure blood pressure by auscultation (Figure 5-13).

With the patient's arm extended with the palm up, place the cuff so that it lies across the upper arm and is located with its distal edge about 1" above the crease at the inside of the patient's elbow. Make sure the center of the inflatable bladder, which is usually marked by an arrow on the cuff, lies over the brachial artery. Next, wrap the ends so that the cuff surrounds the upper arm snugly but not tightly. Secure the cuff with the Velcro fastener attached to it, making sure to rub your hand over the entire area where the two sides of the Velcro fastener are in contact. Once the cuff has been properly secured around the upper arm, the arm should be held at about the same level as the heart.

Next, palpate the brachial artery in the antecubital fossa, located at the anterior aspect of the elbow. Place the diaphragm of the stethoscope over the artery, and hold it firmly pressed against the artery with the fingers of your nondominant hand. Hold the rubber ball-pump in the palm of your other hand and the turn-valve between your thumb and first finger. Close the valve tightly, and pump the ball-pump until the gauge indicates that you have reached a pressure of 200 mm Hg. You should hear no pulse sounds. Slowly turn the valve, opening it until air is steadily escaping from the cuff and you see the hand of the gauge slowly drop. Watch the gauge, and listen carefully. Note the patient's systolic pressure as the reading on the gauge at which the "taps" or "thumps" of the pulse waves can first be heard clearly. As the pressure in the cuff is progressively reduced, pulse sounds will continue for a time, then suddenly disappear. Note the patient's diastolic pressure as the reading on the gauge at which the sounds stopped. At the point at which the sound disappears, the pressure that is exerted against the artery is less than the diastolic pressure. When a greater pressure than the patient's systolic pressure is applied against the outside of the arterial wall, blood flow distal to that point will be occluded, and you will not be able to palpate a distal pulse.

As soon as the pulse sounds stop, open the valve, and release the remaining air quickly. Once you have finished measuring the blood pressure, you should document your findings, the time at which the blood pressure was taken, and in which arm it was taken. Blood pressure is most often measured by auscultation with the

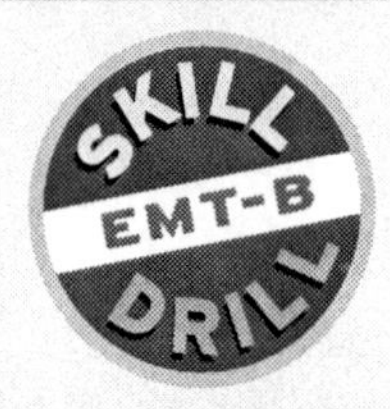

Obtaining a Blood Pressure by Auscultation

Figure 5-13

1

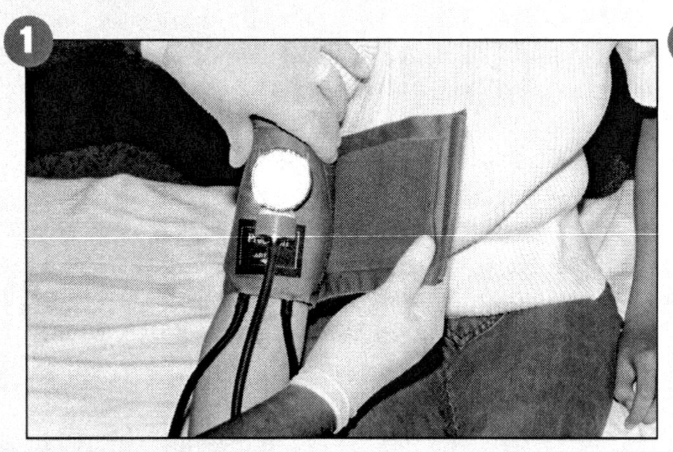

Wrap the cuff snugly around the upper arm, about 1" above the elbow.

2

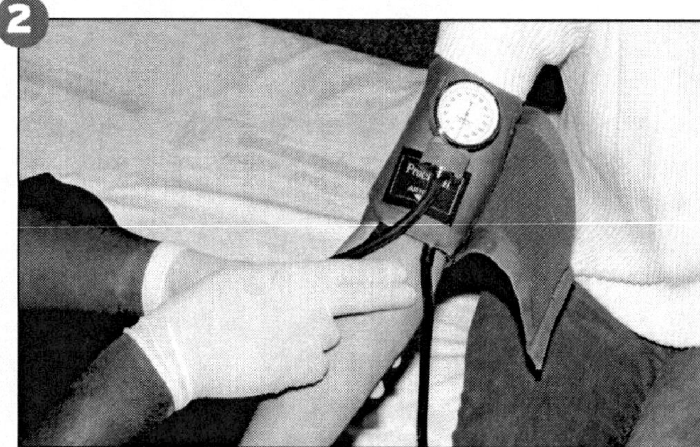

Palpate the brachial pulse to determine where to place the end of the stethoscope.

3

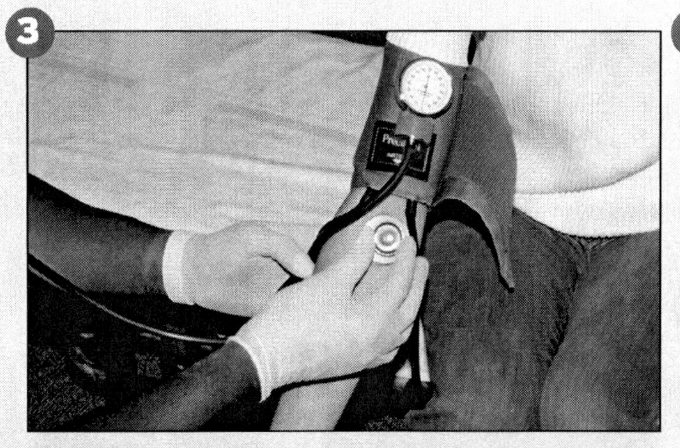

Place the stethoscope over the artery as you hold the ball-pump in your other hand and the turn-valve between your thumb and index finger.

4

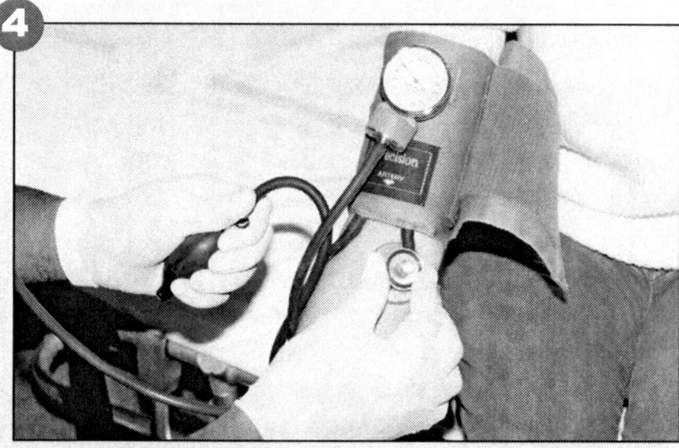

Close the valve, and pump the ball-pump until the gauge reaches 200 mm Hg. At this point, you should hear no sounds. Slowly open the valve until air is steadily escaping from the cuff and you see the pressure dropping. Note the systolic pressure as the reading on the gauge at which you first clearly hear the taps or thumps of the pulse waves. As you continue to release air, the pulse sound will continue for a time and suddenly disappear. Note the diastolic pressure as the reading on the gauge at which the sound stops.

5

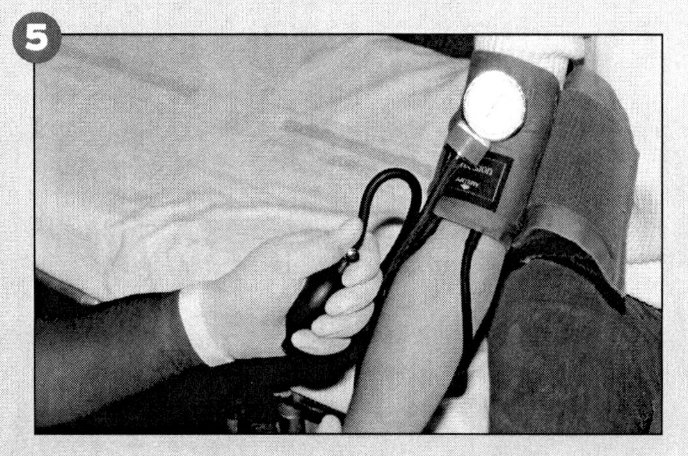

As soon as the sounds stop, open the valve, and release the air quickly.

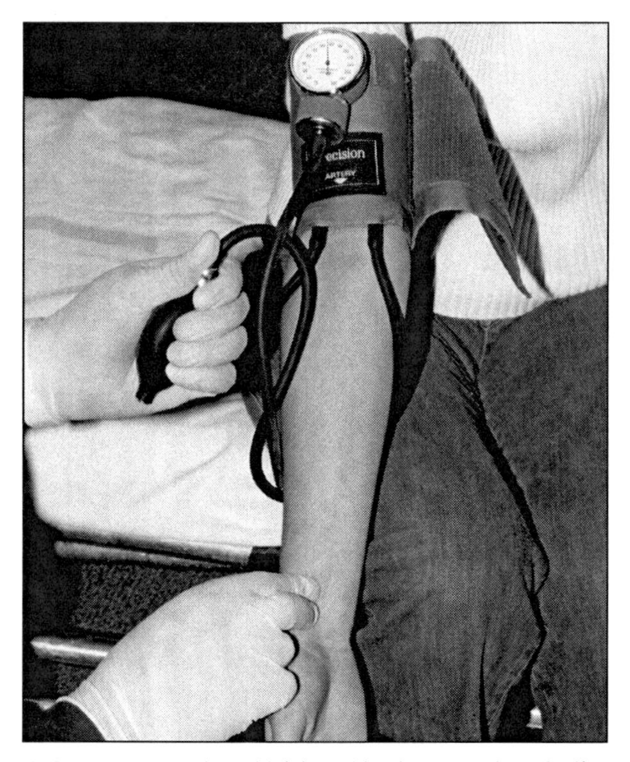

FIGURE 5-14 When obtaining a blood pressure by palpation, you should place your fingertips on the radial artery so that you feel the radial pulse. As you inflate the cuff, you will no longer feel the pulse. Open the turn-valve so that air slowly escapes from the cuff, and watch the gauge. When you can feel the radial pulse again, note the reading on the gauge as the patient's systolic blood pressure.

TABLE 5-4 Normal Ranges for Blood Pressure

Age	Range
Adults	90 to 140 mm Hg (systolic) 60 to 90 mm Hg (diastolic)
Children (ages 1 to 8 years)	80 to 110 mm Hg (systolic)
Infants (newborn to age 1 year)	Two times the patient's age, plus 80

TABLE 5-5 Normal Systolic Blood Pressures

Adult Men	Add 100 to the patient's age, up to 150 mm Hg
Adult Women	Add 90 to the patient's age, up to 150 mm Hg
Children	Add 80 to 2 times the patient's age in years

patient in a sitting or semi-sitting position. Be sure to note whether a different method or position was used.

Occasionally, when a patient's blood pressure is very low, you will continue to hear pulse sounds from the reading at which they started all the way until the gauge has reached 0. When this occurs, you should record the diastolic pressure "0" or "all the way down" to indicate that it was not measurable by stethoscope.

Palpation. The auscultation method will be difficult or impossible to use in a very noisy environment and may produce inaccurate findings. The palpation method, which is examination by touch that does not depend on your ability to hear sounds, should be used in these cases.

To measure blood pressure by palpation, secure the appropriately sized cuff around the patient's upper arm in the manner previously described. With your non-dominant hand, palpate the patient's radial pulse on the same arm as the cuff, without moving your fingertips once you have located it, until you have completed taking the blood pressure (Figure 5-14). While holding the ball-pump in your other hand, close the turn-valve and rapidly inflate the cuff to 200 mm Hg. As the cuff inflates, you will no longer feel the pulse under your fingertips. Open the turn-valve so that air slowly escapes from the cuff, and carefully observe the gauge. When you can again feel the radial pulse under your fingertips, you should note the reading on the gauge as the patient's systolic blood pressure. You will not be able to determine the diastolic pressure with this method. Next, open the turn-valve further, and completely deflate the cuff. Document your findings, including the time and in which arm blood pressure was measured, and note that the pressure was taken by palpation. If you are noting the blood pressure in a box on your run form, you can abbreviate it to "120/by palp."

Normal blood pressure. Blood pressure levels vary with age and gender. Table 5-4 serves as a guideline of normal blood pressure ranges.

A patient has hypotension when the blood pressure is lower than the normal range and hypertension when the blood pressure is higher than the normal range.

Typically, you will see children less frequently than adults; therefore, you might not remember the normal ranges for the various age groups. You might wish to carry a chart in the ambulance and carry-in kit that lists normal blood pressure ranges and other vital sign ranges. Table 5-5 shows rules of thumb that you can also use as a guideline to determine what a patient's systolic pressure should be.

AVPU scale

The AVPU scale is a rapid method of assessing the patient's level of consciousness using one of the following four terms:

A Awake and Alert

V Responsive to Verbal Stimulus

P Responsive to Pain

U Unresponsive

You should determine whether a patient who is awake and alert is oriented to person, place, time, and event. A patient who is oriented will know his or her first and last name. A young child will know his or her first name and whom he or she lives with. A patient who is oriented to place will know his or her location. Most patients who are oriented to time will know the year, month, and day. A patient who is oriented to event will know what happened.

In your report, you can note a person who is oriented to person, place, time, and event as "alert and oriented times four" (A & O x 4). If the patient is not oriented to all four conditions, be sure to note which condition(s) the patient is not oriented to.

A patient who is not awake and alert but who is aroused and responds to your voice by opening his or her eyes, moaning, speaking, or moving is responding to verbal stimulus. A patient who does not respond to your normal speaking voice but who responds to your yelled voice is responding to loud verbal stimulus. Be sure to note how the patient responded. Tap a patient who is hearing impaired with your fingers repeatedly. If the patient responds, note that the patient is hearing impaired but responds to being tapped.

To determine whether a patient who does not respond to verbal stimuli will respond to a painful stimulus, you should gently but firmly pinch the patient's skin (Figure 5-15). A patient who moans or withdraws is responding to painful stimulus. Be sure to note the type and location of the stimulus and how the patient responded.

If the patient does not respond to a painful stimulus on one side, try to elicit a response on the other side. Note that a patient who remains flaccid without moving or making a sound is unresponsive.

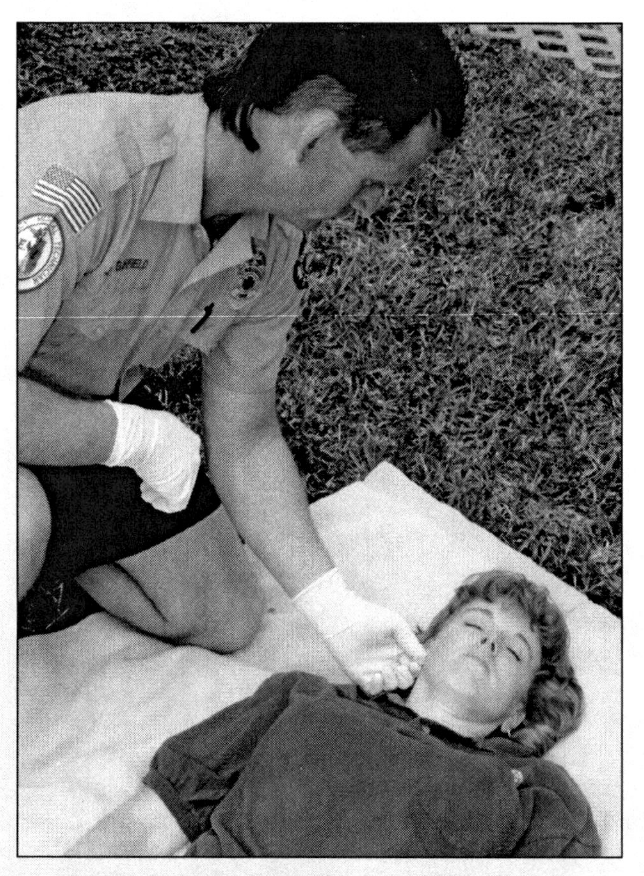

FIGURE 5-15 To assess whether a patient will respond to a painful stimulus, gently, but firmly, pinch the patient's skin. This can be done at the neck or on the earlobe.

TABLE 5-6 Critically Low Systolic Blood Pressures

Male Adults/Adolescents	90 mm Hg or less
Female Adults/Adolescents	80 mm Hg or less
Children	70 mm Hg or less

Critical hypotension. You must assume that a patient who has a critically low blood pressure can no longer compensate sufficiently to maintain adequate perfusion. Table 5-6 shows the point at which blood pressure is considered to be critically low.

In assessing the patient's general circulation, the blood pressure, pulse, skin temperature, and capillary refill should *not* be assessed in an injured limb. However, once you have obtained these vital signs from an uninjured limb, you might wish to compare the distal skin temperature, quality of the distal pulse, and/or capillary refill time in the injured limb with those found on the uninjured side. This information is useful in evaluating whether the injury may have compromised the circulation in the injured limb.

Level of Consciousness

The patient's level of consciousness (LOC) is considered a vital sign because the status of the respiratory, cardiovascular, and central nervous systems are reflected by it. However, in the early assessment, you need to ascertain only the apparent gross level of consciousness by determining whether the patient is awake and alert with an unaltered LOC, conscious but with an altered LOC, or unconscious.

As you assess a patient, you must determine the appropriateness of a response by how well it demonstrates the patient's understanding and mental activity, not how well it reflects your definition of socially acceptable behavior.

When a patient is conscious with a lower level of consciousness, the body's defense mechanisms may no longer be able to compensate adequately, possibly indicating that inadequate perfusion and oxygenation or a chemical or neurologic problem is adversely affecting the brain and its ability to function. A lowered level of consciousness in a conscious patient can also be caused by medications, drugs, alcohol, or poisoning.

Your assessment of a patient who is unconscious when you arrive should be focused initially on ABC and then on identifying other emergency care that the patient may need. Sustained unconsciousness should warn you that a critical respiratory, circulatory, or central nervous system problem or deficit may exist, and you must assume that the patient has a potentially critical injury or condition. In addition, you must consider the condition of any patient who remains unconscious for a sustained period as grave. Therefore, after rapidly assessing the patient and providing any emergency treatment, you should package the patient and provide prompt transport to the hospital.

The Glasgow Coma Scale is a method of assessing a patient's level of consciousness by scoring the patient's response to eye opening, motor response, and verbal response (Figure 5-16).

GLASGOW COMA SCALE

Eye Opening		
Spontaneous	4	
To Voice	3	
To Pain	2	
None	1	
Verbal Response		
Oriented	5	
Confused	4	
Inappropriate Words	3	
Incomprehensible Words	2	
None	1	
Motor Response		
Obeys Command	6	
Localizes Pain	5	
Withdraws (pain)	4	
Flexion (pain)	3	
Extension (pain)	2	
None	1	
Glasgow Coma Score Total	**15**	

FIGURE 5-16 The Glasgow Coma Scale.

Pupils. The diameter of the patient's pupils reflects the status of the brain's perfusion, oxygenation, and condition (Figure 5-17). The pupil is a circular opening in the center of the pigmented iris of the eye. The pupils are normally round and of approximately equal size and serve as optical diaphragms, adjusting their size depending on the available light. In normal room light, the pupil appears to be midsize. With less light, the pupils dilate, allowing more light to enter the eye, making it possible to see even in dim light. With high light levels or when a bright light is suddenly introduced, the pupils instantly constrict, allowing less light to enter, protecting the sensitive receptors in the inner eye from damage. When a brighter light is introduced into one eye (or higher levels of light enter one eye only), both pupils should constrict equally to the appropriate size for the pupil receiving the most light.

In the absence of any light, the pupils will become fully relaxed and dilated. When light is introduced, each eye sends sensory signals to the brain indicating the level of light it is receiving. Pupil size is regulated by a series of continuous motor commands that the brain automatically sends through the oculomotor nerves to each eye, causing both pupils to constrict to the same appropriate size. Normally, pupil size changes instantly to any change in light level.

You must assume the patient has depressed brain function as a result of either central nervous system depression or injury if the pupils react in any of the following ways:

- Become fixed with no reaction to light
- Dilate with introduction of a bright light and constrict when the light is removed
- React sluggishly instead of briskly
- Become unequal in size
- Become unequal in size when a bright light is introduced into or removed from one eye

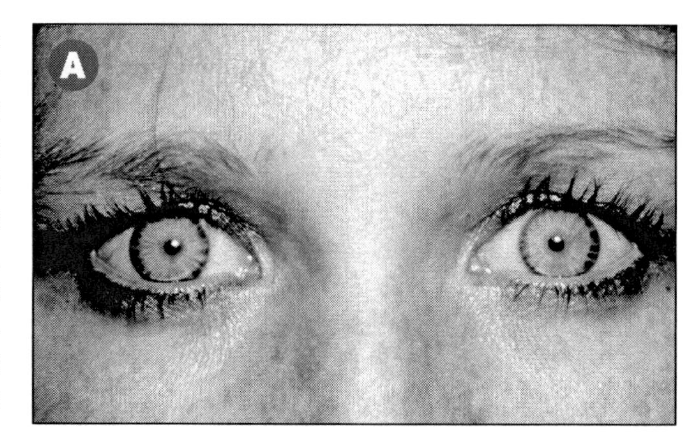

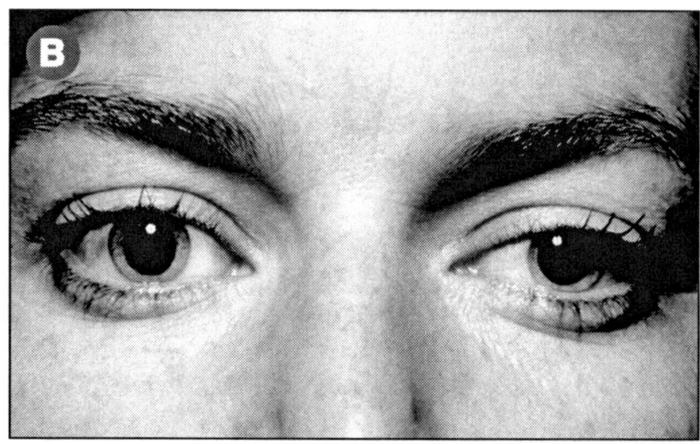

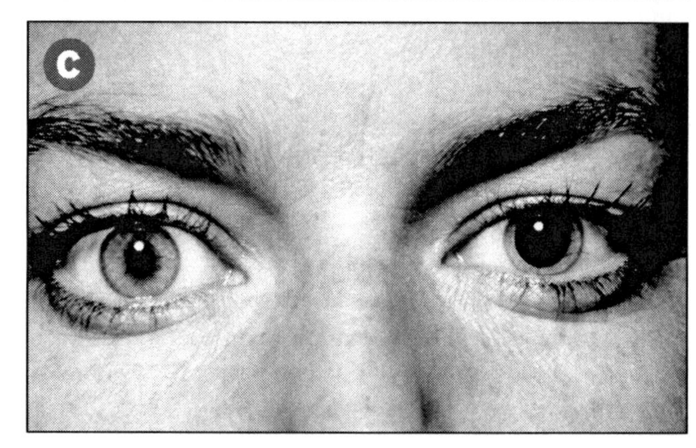

FIGURE 5-17 **A:** Constricted pupils. **B:** Dilated pupils. **C:** Unequal pupils.

Depressed brain function can be produced by the following situations:

- Injury of the brain or brain stem
- Trauma or stroke
- Brain tumor or other growth
- Inadequate oxygenation or perfusion
- Drugs or toxins (central nervous system depressants)

Opiates, which are one category of central nervous system depressants, cause the pupils to constrict so significantly, regardless of light, that they become so small as to be described as pinpoint. Intracranial pressure from intracranial bleeding at the side of the head may cause sufficient pressure against the oculomotor nerve on one side that the motor commands can no longer pass from the brain to that eye. When this occurs, the eye no longer receives commands to constrict, and its pupil becomes fully dilated and fixed. This is described as a blown pupil.

Pupils may be dilated, may be unequal as a result of medication placed into one or both eyes or from an injury or condition of the eye, or may not be reacting appropriately. You cannot determine the cause as you assess the patient. Further examination of the patient in the emergency department will determine the cause.

The letters PEARRL serve as a useful guide in assessing the pupils. They stand for the following:

P = **P**upils

E = **E**qual

A = **A**nd

R = **R**ound

R = **R**egular in size

L = react to **L**ight

You can report patients with normal pupils as "Pupils are equal, round, and regular in size, and react properly to light" or "the patient has PEARRL." Describe any abnormal findings using the longer form, such as "Pupils are equal and round, the left pupil is dilated and fixed, the right pupil is regular in size and reacts to light."

Reassessment of the Vital Signs

The vital signs that you obtain serve two important functions. The first set establishes an important initial measurement of the patient's respiratory and cardiovascular systems and the quality of perfusion and oxygenation of the brain and other vital organs. The initial vital signs also serve as a key baseline.

Throughout your care of the patient, you should monitor the patient's vital signs for any changes from your initial findings. You should reassess and record vital signs at least every 15 minutes in a stable patient and at least every 5 minutes in an unstable patient. You should also reassess and record vital signs following all medical interventions. This ongoing comparative assessment is an important indicator of whether your interventions have restored the patient's vital functions to an acceptable range or are at least preventing further deterioration. Reassessment also indicates whether you should consider more aggressive intervention whenever deterioration continues.

You should reassess and record vital signs at least every 15 minutes in a stable patient and at least every 5 minutes in an unstable patient.

Obtaining a SAMPLE History

Once you have provided emergency care and are ready to further examine the patient, you should try to obtain a key brief history, or SAMPLE history. As part of the assessment of every patient, you should ask the following questions, using the word SAMPLE as a guideline:

- **S**igns and **S**ymptoms of the episode: What signs and symptoms occurred at onset of the incident? Does the patient report pain? If so, where is the pain and how strong is it on a scale of 1 to 10? How often does the pain occur and how long does it last?
- **A**llergies: Is the patient allergic to any medication, food, or other substance? What reactions did the patient have to any of them? If the patient has no known allergies, you should note this on the run report as "no known allergies" or "nka."
- **M**edications: What medications was the patient prescribed? What dosage was prescribed? How often is the patient supposed to take the medication? What prescription and over-the-counter medications has the patient taken in the last 12 hours? How much was taken and when?
- **P**ertinent past history: Does the patient have any history of medical, surgical, or trauma occurrences? Has the patient had a recent accident, fall, blow to the head? Was the patient unconscious at any time before or since the incident occurred?
- **L**ast oral intake: When did the patient last eat or drink? What did the patient eat or drink and how much was consumed? Did the patient take any drugs or drink alcohol? Has there been any other oral intake in the last 4 hours?
- **E**vents leading to the injury or illness: What are the key events that led up to this incident? What occurred between the onset of the incident and your arrival? Has the patient experienced any chest pain? If so, did it occur during exertion or while the patient was at rest?

With practice, you will be able to obtain, document, and report a meaningful brief history. Be sure to ask the patient and bystanders for information. If the patient is unconscious, look for a medical identification tag or for a medical information card in the patient's wallet or purse. *Always* look for patient identification in the presence of another EMT or law enforcement officer at the scene.

prep kit

ready for review

Whenever you are called to the scene of an illness or injury, you should find out the patient's chief complaint. Your assessment of the patient should include rapidly evaluating the patient's general condition and identifying any potentially life-threatening injuries or conditions. Baseline vital signs are the key signs that you will use to evaluate the patient's general condition. You will be assessing the patient's respirations, pulse, skin, capillary refill, blood pressure, level of consciousness, and pupils.

After you have initially assessed the patient and obtained the baseline vital signs, you should reassess the patient for any changes from your initial findings.

In addition to determining the chief complaint and assessing the patient's general condition, you should try to obtain a SAMPLE history from the patient or bystanders. By asking several important questions, you will be able to determine the patient's signs and symptoms, allergies, medications taken, pertinent past history, last oral intake, and the events leading up to the incident.

vital vocabulary

www.emtb.com

auscultation A method of listening to sounds within an organ with a stethoscope.

AVPU scale A method of assessing a patient's level of consciousness by determining whether the patient is awake and alert, responsive to verbal stimulus or pain, or unresponsive; used principally in the initial assessment.

blood pressure (BP) The pressure of circulating blood against the walls of the arteries.

bradycardia Slow heart rate, less than 60 beats/min.

capillary refill A test that evaluates the ability of the circulatory system to restore blood to the capillary system.

chief complaint The reason a patient called for help. Also, the patient's response to questions such as "What's wrong?" or "What happened?"

cyanosis A bluish, gray skin color that is caused by reduced levels of oxygen in the blood.

diastolic pressure The component of blood pressure in which pressure remains in the arteries during the relaxing phase of the heart's cycle when the left ventricle is at rest.

Glasgow Coma Scale A method of assessing a patient's level of consciousness by scoring the patient's response to eye opening, motor response, and verbal response; used primarily in the detailed and ongoing assessment.

hypertension Blood pressure that is higher than the normal range.

hypotension Blood pressure that is lower than the normal range.

jaundice A yellow skin color that is caused by liver disease or dysfunction.

labored breathing A way in which to describe breathing that requires increased effort; characterized by grunting, stridor, and use of accessory muscles.

perfusion Circulation of blood within an organ or tissue in adequate amounts to meet the cells' current needs.

pulse The pressure wave that occurs as each heartbeat causes a surge in the blood circulating through the arteries.

SAMPLE history A key brief history of a patient's condition to determine signs and symptoms, allergies, medications, pertinent past history, last oral intake, and events leading to the injury or illness.

sign An objective finding that can be seen, heard, felt, smelled, or measured.

sniffing position An unusually upright position in which the patient's head and chin are thrust slightly forward; also called a tripod position.

spontaneous respirations Breathing in a patient that occurs with no assistance.

stridor A harsh, high-pitched inspiratory sound, such as the sound often heard in acute laryngeal (upper airway) obstruction.

symptom A subjective finding that the patient feels but that can be identified only by the patient.

systolic pressure The component of blood pressure in which pressure is increased along an artery with each contraction of the ventricle.

tachycardia Rapid heart rhythm, more than 100 beats/min.

tidal volume The amount of air that is exchanged with each breath.

vital signs The key signs that are used to evaluate the patient's overall condition, including respirations, pulse, blood pressure, level of consciousness, and skin characteristics.

assessment in action

You and your partner are dispatched to a private residence, where you find a 63-year-old woman complaining that she is "dizzy and weak everywhere" and that she has felt this way for almost three weeks. The patient is alert and oriented but looks angry. She demands to know why it took you so long to respond. The patient says that she has no allergies and takes no medications other than an aspirin every day. Your partner obtains baseline vital signs as you interview the patient. She has a blood pressure of 148/82 mm Hg, a regular pulse of 92 beats/min, respirations of 16/min, and warm, dry skin.

1. The "A" in the SAMPLE history refers to:
   A. Age.
   B. Affect.
   C. Attitude.
   D. Allergies.
2. The "M" in the SAMPLE history refers to:
   A. Medications.
   B. Mental status.
   C. Motor response.
   D. Memories of yesterday.
3. The "P" in the SAMPLE history refers to:
   A. Pulse checks.
   B. Pupil status response.
   C. Possible diagnosis.
   D. Past pertinent events.
4. The "L" in the SAMPLE history refers to:
   A. Life history.
   B. Last oral intake.
   C. Length of illness.
   D. Level of consciousness.
5. The "E" in the SAMPLE history refers to:
   A. Ear, nose or throat problems.
   B. Events leading up to the illness or injury.
   C. Exercises that the patient does.
   D. Estimated time since the symptoms started.

points to ponder

Objectives 1-5.28, 1-5.31, 1-1.8, 1-3.9

You have responded to a 34-year-old patient who was in-line skating and fell. The patient has scrapes on both knees and is bleeding from an open fracture of the left ulna. While controlling the bleeding, you begin asking SAMPLE history questions. When you ask about pertinent past history, the patient tells you that he is HIV positive but asks you not to tell anyone. The patient is currently quite healthy and does not want others to know. The patient is also afraid that if you tell the hospital, his insurance carrier will find out.

- Would you record this information and/or pass it on to the hospital? Why or why not?

online outlook

If time permits, you should attempt to learn the patient's SAMPLE history. Improve your ability to identify SAMPLE information by completing Exercise 5 at www.emtb.com.

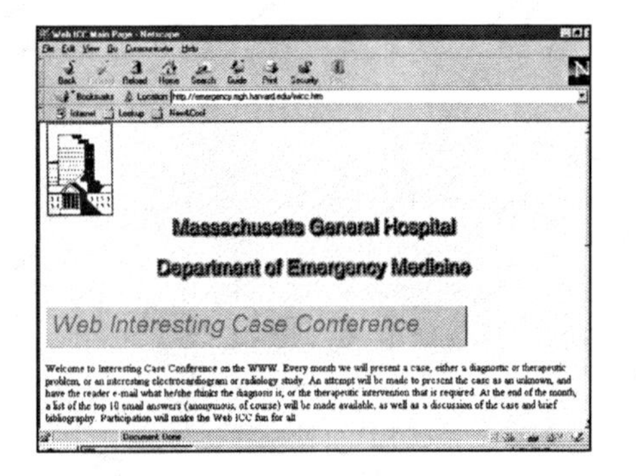

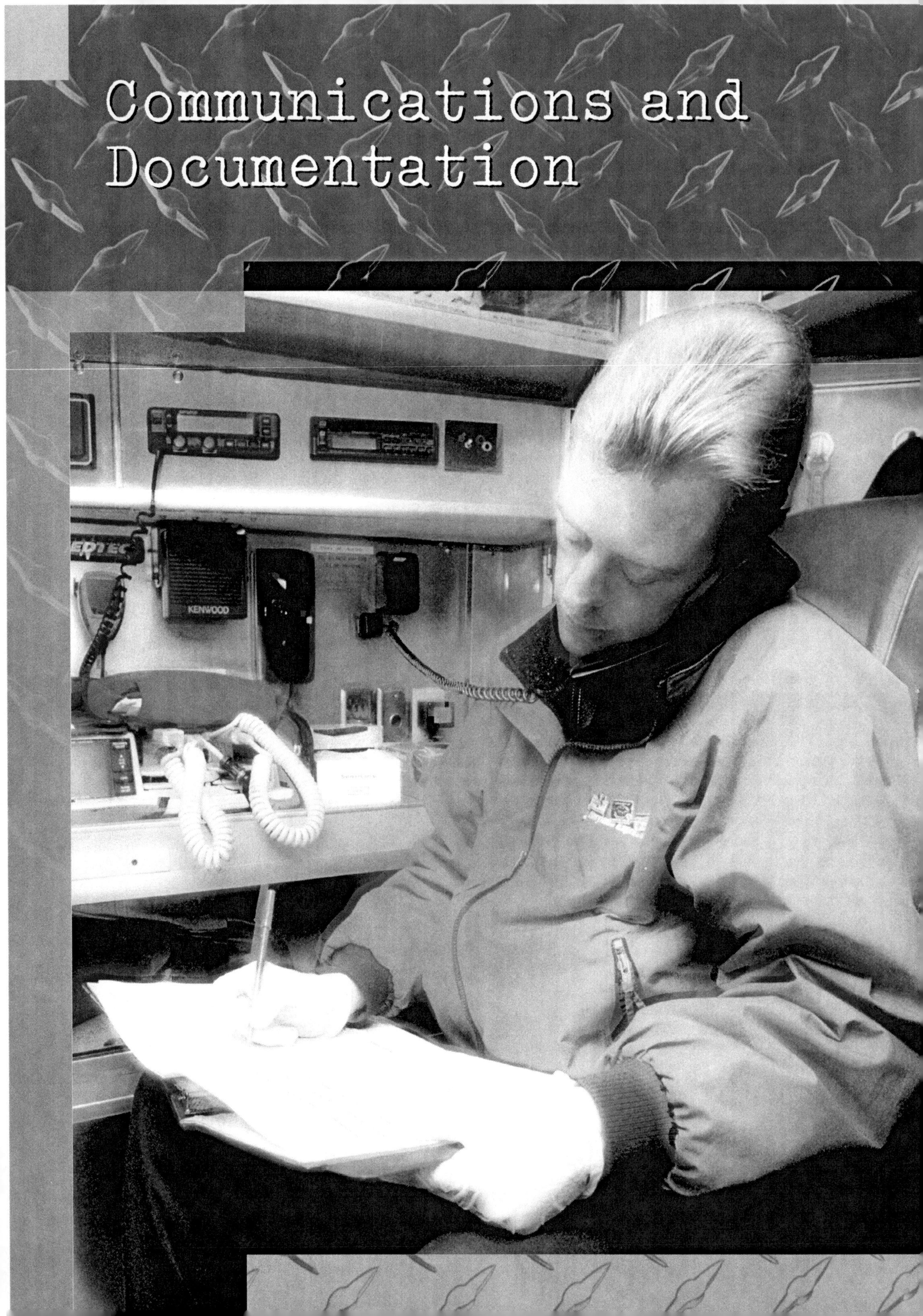
Communications and
Documentation
KENWOOD

chapter 3

objectives

Cognitive

1. List the proper methods of initiating and terminating a radio call.
2. State the proper sequence for delivery of patient information.
3. Explain the importance of effective communication of patient information in the verbal report.
4. Identify the essential components of the verbal report.
5. Describe the attributes for increasing effectiveness and efficiency of verbal communications.
6. State legal aspects to consider in verbal communication.
7. Discuss the communication skills that should be used to interact with the patient.
8. Discuss the communication skills that should be used to interact with the family, bystanders, individuals from other agencies while providing patient care and hospital personnel, and the difference between skills used to interact with the patient and those used to interact with others.
9. List the correct radio procedures in the following phases of a typical call:
   - To the scene
   - At the scene
   - To the facility
   - At the facility
   - To the station
   - At the station
10. Explain the components of the written report and list the information that should be included on the written report.
11. Identify the various sections of the written report.
12. Describe what information is required in each section of the prehospital care report and how it should be entered.
13. Define the special considerations concerning patient refusal.
14. Describe the legal implications associated with the written report.
15. Discuss all state and/or local record and reporting requirements.

Affective

16. Explain the rationale for providing efficient and effective radio communications and patient reports.
17. Explain the rationale for patient care documentation.
18. Explain the rationale for the EMS system gathering data.
19. Explain the rationale for using medical terminology correctly.
20. Explain the rationale for using an accurate and synchronous clock so that information can be used in trending.

Psychomotor

21. Perform a simulated, organized, concise radio transmission.
22. Perform an organized, concise patient report that would be given to the staff at a receiving facility.
23. Perform a brief, organized report that would be given to an ALS provider arriving at an incident scene at which the EMT-B was already providing care.
24. Practice completing a prehospital care report.

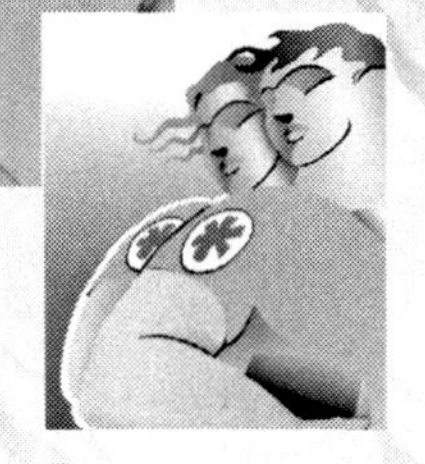

you are the cfr/emt

You reach for your portable radio to contact the base station for orders, but you realize that it is gone! To complicate matters, you and your partner are alone at the bottom of a ravine working a motor vehicle crash with three patients.

Given the adverse circumstances in which you will often find yourself working, something of this nature may happen to you. This chapter will introduce you to medical communications and documentation. It will also help you to answer the following questions:

1. What is the appropriate course of action in the situation described above? What happens when you have lost the ability to communicate with the hospital?
2. What are the advantages and disadvantages of using narrative-style run reports compared with "fill-in-the-bubble" style reports?

Communications and Documentation

Effective communication is an essential component of prehospital care. Radio and telephone communications link you and your team with other members of the EMS, fire, and law enforcement communities. This link helps the entire team to work together more effectively and provides an important layer of safety and protection for each member of the team. You must know what your system can and cannot do, and you must be able to use your system efficiently and effectively. You must be able to send precise, accurate reports about the scene, the patient's condition, and the treatment that you provide.

Verbal communications are also a vital skill for EMT-Bs. Your verbal skills will enable you to gather information from the patient and bystanders. They will also make it possible for you to effectively coordinate the variety of responders who are often present at the scene. Excellent verbal communications are also an integral part of transferring the patient's care to the nurses and physicians at the hospital. You must possess good listening skills to fully understand the nature of the scene and the patient's problem. You must also be able to organize your thoughts to quickly and accurately verbalize instructions to the patient, bystanders, and other responders. Finally, you must be able to organize and summarize the important aspects of the patient's presentation and treatment when reporting to the hospital staff.

Written communications complete the process. Written communications, in the form of a written patient care report, provide you with an opportunity to communicate the patient's story to others who may participate in the patient's care in the future. Adequate reporting and accurate records ensure the continuity of patient care. Complete patient records also guarantee proper transfer of responsibility, comply with the requirements of health departments and law enforcement agencies, and fulfill your organization's administrative needs. Reporting and record-keeping duties are an essential aspect of patient care, although they must be performed only after the patient's condition has been stabilized.

This chapter describes the skills that you need to be an effective communicator. It begins by identifying the kinds of equipment that are used, along with standard radio operating procedures and protocols. Next, the roles of the Federal Communications Commission (FCC) in EMS are described. The chapter concludes with a discussion of a variety of effective methods of verbal communications and guidelines for appropriate written documentation of patient care.

Communications Systems and Equipment

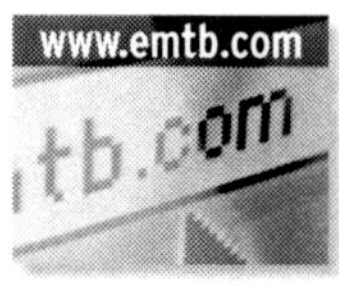

As an EMT-B, you must be familiar with two-way radio communications and have working knowledge of the mobile and hand-held portable radios that are used in your unit. You must also know when to use them and what to say when you are transmitting.

Base Station Radios

The dispatcher usually communicates with field units by transmitting through a fixed radio base station that is controlled from the dispatch center. A base station is any radio hardware containing a transmitter and receiver that is located in a fixed place (Figure 9-1). The base station may be used in a single place by an operator speaking into a microphone that is connected directly to the equipment. It also works remotely through telephone lines or by radio from a communications center. Base stations may include dispatch centers, fire stations, ambulance bases, or hospitals.

A two-way radio consists of two units: a transmitter and a receiver. Some base stations may have more than one transmitter and/or more than one receiver. They may also be equipped with one multi-channel transmitter and several single channel receivers. A channel is an assigned frequency or frequencies that are used to carry voice and/or data communications. Regardless of the number of transmitters and receivers, they are commonly called base radios or stations. Base stations usually have more power (often 100 watts or more) and higher, more efficient antenna systems than mobile or portable radios. This increased broadcasting range allows the base station operator to communicate with field units and other stations at much greater distances.

The base radio must be physically close to its antenna. Therefore, the actual base station cabinet and hardware are commonly found on the roof of a tall building or at the bottom of an antenna tower. The base station operator may be miles away in a dispatch center or hospital, communicating with the base station radio by dedicated lines or special radio links.

A two-way radio consists of two units: a transmitter and a receiver.

A dedicated line, also known as a hot line, is always open or under the control of the individuals at each end. This type of line is immediately "on" as soon as you lift the receiver and cannot be accessed by outside users.

Mobile and Portable Radios

In the ambulance, you will use both mobile and portable radios to communicate with the dispatcher and/or medical control. An ambulance will often have more than one mobile radio, each on a different frequency (Figure 9-2). One radio may be used to communicate with the dispatcher or other public safety agencies. A second radio is often used for communicating patient information to medical control.

A mobile radio is installed in a vehicle and usually operates at lower power than a base station. Most VHF (very high frequency) mobile radios operate at 100 watts of power. Radios that operate at 800 MHz of power are very common in EMS systems. UHF (ultra-high frequency) mobile radios usually have only 40 watts of power. Cellular telephones operate on 3 watts of power or less. Mobile antennas are much closer to the ground than base station antennas, so communications from the unit are typically limited to 10 to 15 miles over average terrain.

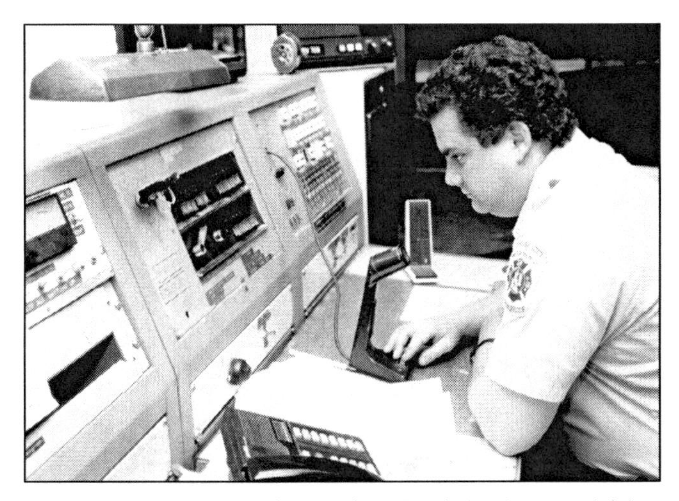

FIGURE 9-1 A base station consists of radio hardware containing a transmitter and a receiver that is located in a fixed place. Some have more than one transmitter and/or more than one receiver.

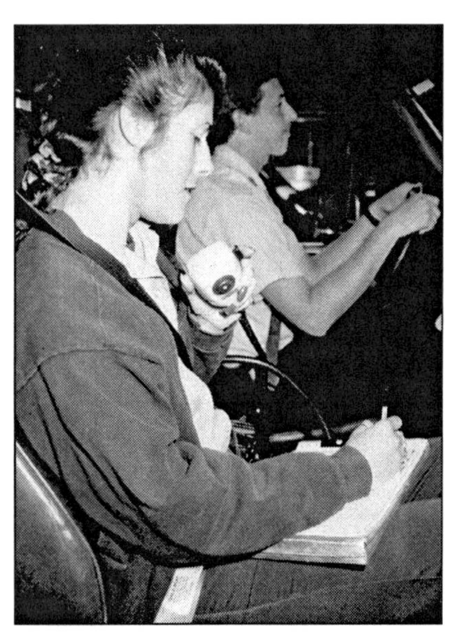

FIGURE 9-2 Some ambulances have more than one mobile radio, each on a different frequency.

Portable radios are hand-carried or hand-held devices that operate at 1 to 5 watts of power (Figure 9-3). Since the entire radio can be held in your hand, when in use the antenna is often no higher than the EMT who is using the radio. The transmission range of a portable radio is more limited than that of mobile or base station radios. Portable radios are essential in helping to coordinate EMS activities at the scene of a multiple-casualty incident. They are also helpful when you are away from the ambulance and need to communicate with dispatch, another unit, or medical control.

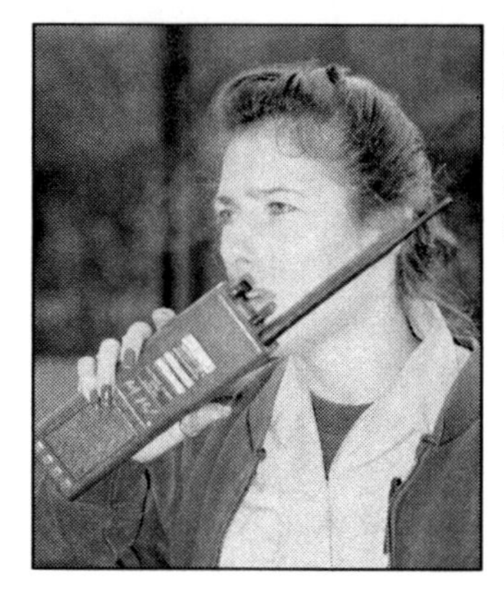

FIGURE 9-3 A portable radio is essential if you need to communicate with the dispatcher or medical control when you are away from the ambulance.

Repeater-Based Systems

A repeater is a special base station radio that receives messages and signals on one frequency and then automatically retransmits them on a second frequency. Because a repeater is a base station (with a large antenna), it is able to receive lower-power signals, such as those from a portable radio, from a long distance away. The signal is then rebroadcast with all the power of the base station (Figure 9-4). EMS systems that use repeaters usually have outstanding system-wide communications and are able to get the best signal from portable radios.

Digital Equipment

Although most people think of voice communications when they think of two-way radios, digital signals are also a part of EMS communications. Some EMS systems use telemetry to send an ECG from the unit to the hospital. With telemetry, electronic signals are converted into coded, audible signals. These signals can then be transmitted by radio or telephone to a receiver at the hospital with a decoder. The decoder converts the signals back into electronic impulses that can be displayed on a screen or printed. Another example of telemetry is a fax message.

Digital signals are also used in some kinds of paging and tone alerting systems because they transmit faster than spoken words and allow more choices and flexibility.

Cellular Telephones

Cellular telephones are becoming more common in EMS communications systems (Figure 9-5). These telephones are simply low-power portable radios that communicate through a series of interconnected repeater stations called "cells" (hence the name "cellular"). Cells are linked by a sophisticated computer system and connected to the telephone network. Cellular telephones are also popular with other public safety agencies, particularly as more cell sites are constructed in rural areas.

Unlike typical two-way mobile communications, which have free access, a cellular system charges fees for its use. Your system can buy portable or mobile radios on the local EMS frequency and use them at no cost. However, buying a cellular telephone is only half of the process of being able to use it. A cellular telephone cannot simply access the telephone network. The user must be assigned a specially coded number that the cellular system's computers will recognize. It is that access and the amount of time a user spends on the telephone for

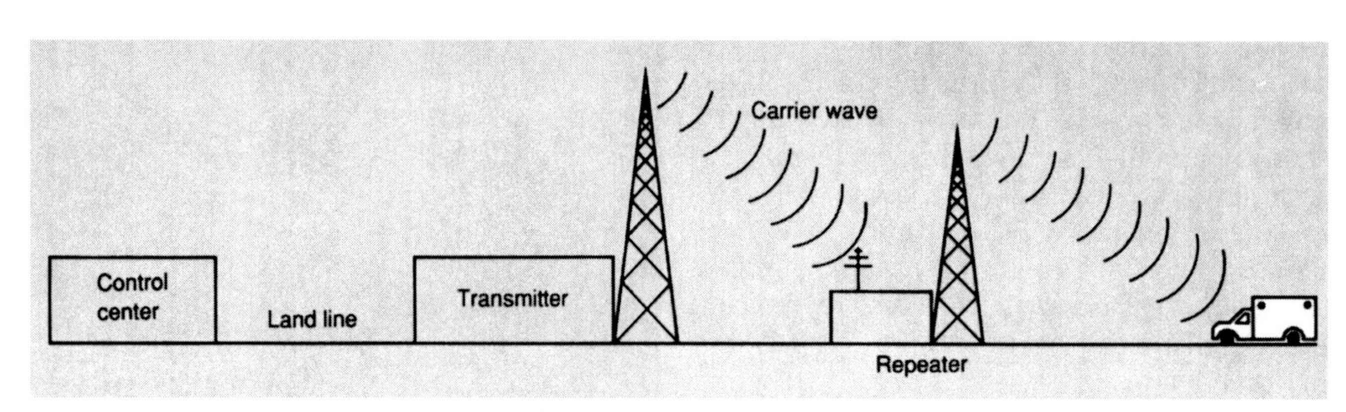

FIGURE 9-4 A message is sent from the control center by a land line to the transmitter. The radio carrier wave is picked up by the repeater for rebroadcast to outlying units. Return radio traffic is picked up by the repeater and rebroadcast to the control center.

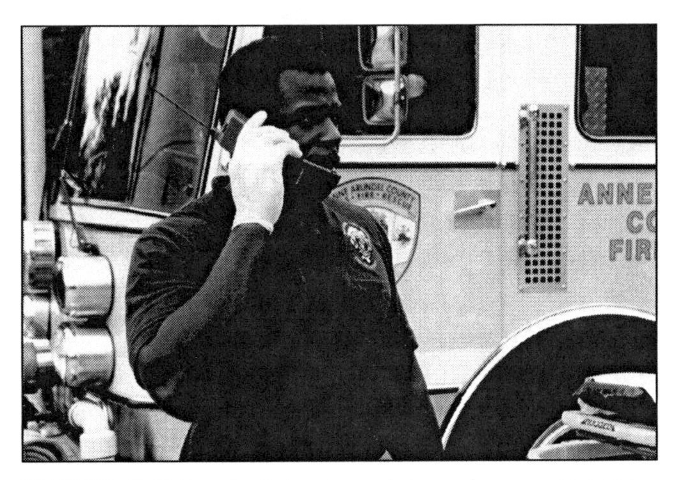

FIGURE 9-5 Use of cellular phones is becoming more common in EMS communications systems.

which the cellular system charges. However, once you are connected to the network, you can call any other telephone in the world and can send voice, data, and telemetry signals.

Many cellular systems make equipment and air time available to EMS services at little or no cost as a public service. The public is often able to call 9-1-1 or other emergency numbers on a cellular telephone free of charge. However, this easy access may result in overloading and jamming of cellular systems in mass-casualty and disaster situations.

As with all repeater-based systems, a cellular telephone is useless if the equipment fails, loses power, or is damaged by severe weather or other circumstances. Like all voice radio communications systems, cellular telephones can be easily overheard on scanners. A scanner is a radio receiver that searches or "scans" across several frequencies until the message is completed. Although cellular telephones are more private than most other forms of radio communications, they can still be overheard. Therefore, you must always speak in a professional manner every time you use the EMS communications system.

Other Communications Equipment

Ambulances and other field units are usually equipped with an external public address system. This system may be a part of the siren or the mobile radio. The intercom between the cab and the patient compartment may also be a part of the mobile radio. These components do not involve radio wave transmission, but you must understand how they work and practice using them *before* you really need them.

EMS systems may use a variety of two-way radio hardware. Some systems operate VHF equipment in the simplex (push to talk, release to listen) mode. In this mode, radio transmissions can occur in either direction but not simultaneously in both. When one party transmits, the other can only receive and then wait for the other party to finish before he or she can reply. Other systems conduct duplex (simultaneous talk-listen) communications on UHF frequencies and also use cellular telephones. In the full duplex mode, radios can transmit and receive communications simultaneously on one channel. This is sometimes called "a pair of frequencies." A number of VHF and UHF channels, commonly called MED channels, are reserved exclusively for EMS use. However, hundreds of other commercial, local government, and fire services frequencies are also used for EMS communications.

Some EMS systems rely on dedicated lines (hot lines) as control links for their remotely located base stations and antennas. Other systems are more simply configured and require no off-site control links. No matter what type of equipment is used, all EMS communications systems have some basic limitations. Therefore, you must know what your equipment can and cannot do.

The ability for you to communicate effectively with other units or medical control depends on how well the weaker radio can "talk back." Base and repeater station radios often have much greater power and higher antennas than mobile or portable units do. This increased power affects your communications in two ways. First, their signals are generally heard and understood from a much greater distance than the signal produced from a mobile unit. Second, their signals are received clearly from a much greater distance than is possible with a mobile or portable unit. *Remember, when you are at the scene, you may be able to clearly hear the dispatcher or hospital on your radio, but you may not be heard or understood when you transmit.*

Even small changes in your location can significantly affect the quality of your transmission. Also remember that the location of the antenna is critically important for clear transmission. Commercial aircraft flying at 37,000' can transmit and receive signals over hundreds of miles, yet their radios have only a few watts of power. The "power" comes from their 37,000-foot-high antenna!

You must always speak in a professional manner every time you use the EMS communications system.

At times, you may be able to communicate with a base station radio but you will not be able to hear or transmit to another mobile unit that is also communicating with that base. Repeater base stations eliminate such problems. They allow two mobile or portable units that cannot reach each other directly to communicate through the repeater, using its greater power and antenna.

The success of communications depends on the efficiency of your equipment. A damaged antenna or microphone often prevents high-quality communications. Check the condition and status of your equipment at the start of each shift, and then correct or report any problems.

Radio Communications

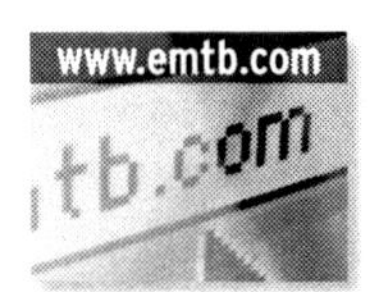

All radio operations in the United States, including those used in EMS systems, are regulated by the Federal Communications Commission (FCC). The FCC has jurisdiction over interstate and international telephone and telegraph services and satellite communications—all of which may involve EMS activity.

The FCC has five principal EMS-related responsibilities:

1. **Allocating specific radio frequencies for use by EMS providers.** Modern EMS communications began in 1974. At that time, the FCC assigned 10 MED channels in the 460- to 470-MHz (UHF) band to be used by EMS providers. These UHF channels were added to the several VHF frequencies that were already available for EMS systems. However, these VHF frequencies had to be shared with other "special emergencies" uses, including school buses and veterinarians. In 1993, the FCC created an EMS-only block of frequencies in the 220-MHz portion of the radio spectrum.
2. **Licensing base stations and assigning appropriate radio call signs for those stations.** An FCC license is usually issued for 5 years, after which time it must be renewed. Each FCC license is granted only for a specific operating group. Often, the longitude and latitude (locations) of the antenna and the address of the base station determine the call signs.
3. **Establishing licensing standards and operating specifications for radio equipment used by EMS providers.** Before it can be licensed, each piece of radio equipment must be submitted by its manufacturer to the FCC for type acceptance, based on established operating specification and regulations.
4. **Establishing limitations for transmitter power output.** The FCC regulates broadcasting power to reduce radio interference between neighboring communications systems.
5. **Monitoring radio operations.** This includes making spot field checks to help ensure compliance with FCC rules and regulations.

The FCC's rules and regulations fill many volumes and are written in technical and legal language. Only a very small section (part 90, subpart C) deals with EMS communication issues. You are not responsible for reading these detailed and often confusing documents. For appropriate guidance on technical issues, contact your EMS system supervisor. In fact, many EMS systems look to radio and telephone communications experts for advice on technical issues.

Responding to the Scene

EMS communication systems may operate on several different frequencies and may use different frequency bands. Some EMS systems may even use different radios for different purposes. However, all EMS systems depend on the skill of the dispatcher. The dispatcher, who is usually not an EMT-B, receives the first call to 9-1-1 (Figure 9-6). You are part of the team that responds to calls once the dispatcher notifies your unit of an emergency.

The dispatcher has several important responsibilities during the alert and dispatch phase of EMS communications. The dispatcher must do all of the following:

- Properly screen and assign priority to each call (according to predetermined protocols)
- Select and alert the appropriate EMS response unit(s)
- Dispatch and direct EMS response unit(s) to the correct location

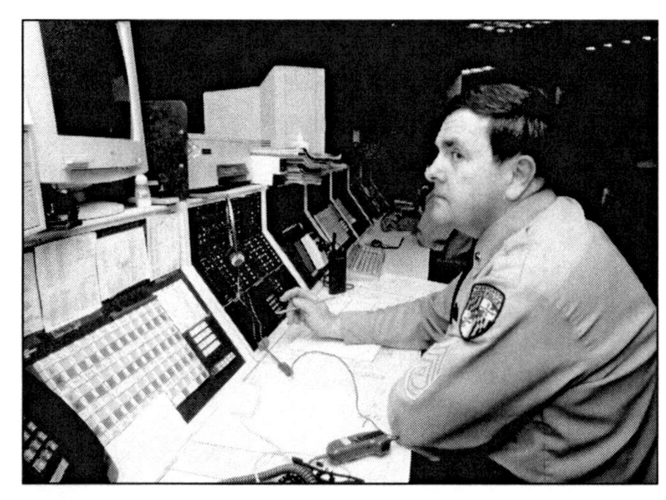

FIGURE 9-6 The dispatcher receives the first call to 9-1-1.

- Coordinate EMS response unit(s) with other public safety services until the incident is over
- Provide emergency medical instructions to the telephone caller so that essential care (e.g., CPR) may begin before the EMTs arrive (according to predetermined protocols).

When the first call to 9-1-1 comes in, the dispatcher must try to judge its relative importance to begin the appropriate EMS response using emergency medical dispatch protocols. First, the dispatcher must find out the exact location of the patient and the nature and severity of the problem. Next, some description of the scene, such as the number of patients or special environmental hazards, is needed. Then, if possible, the dispatcher should ask for the caller's telephone number, the patient's age and name, and other information, as directed by local protocol.

From this information, the dispatcher will assign the appropriate EMS response unit(s) on the basis of the following:

- The dispatcher's perception of the nature and severity of the problem
- The anticipated response time to the scene
- The level of training (first responder, BLS, ALS) of available EMS response unit(s)
- The need for additional EMS units, fire suppression, rescue, a HazMat team, air medical support, or law enforcement

The dispatcher's next step is to alert the appropriate EMS response unit(s) (Figure 9-7). Alerting these units may be done in a variety of ways. The dispatch radio system may be used to contact units that are already in service and monitoring the channel. Dedicated lines (hot lines) between the control center and the EMS station may also be used.

The dispatcher may also page EMS personnel. Pagers are commonly used by both volunteer and full-time EMS personnel. Paging involves the use of a coded tone or digital radio signal and a voice or display message that is transmitted to pagers (beepers) or desktop monitor radios. Paging signals may be sent to alert only certain personnel or may be blanket signals that will activate all the pagers in the EMS service. Pagers and monitor radios are convenient because they are usually silent until their specific paging code is received. Alerted personnel contact the dispatcher to confirm the message and receive details of their assignments.

Once EMS personnel have been alerted, they must be properly dispatched and sent to the incident. Every EMS system should use a standard dispatching procedure.

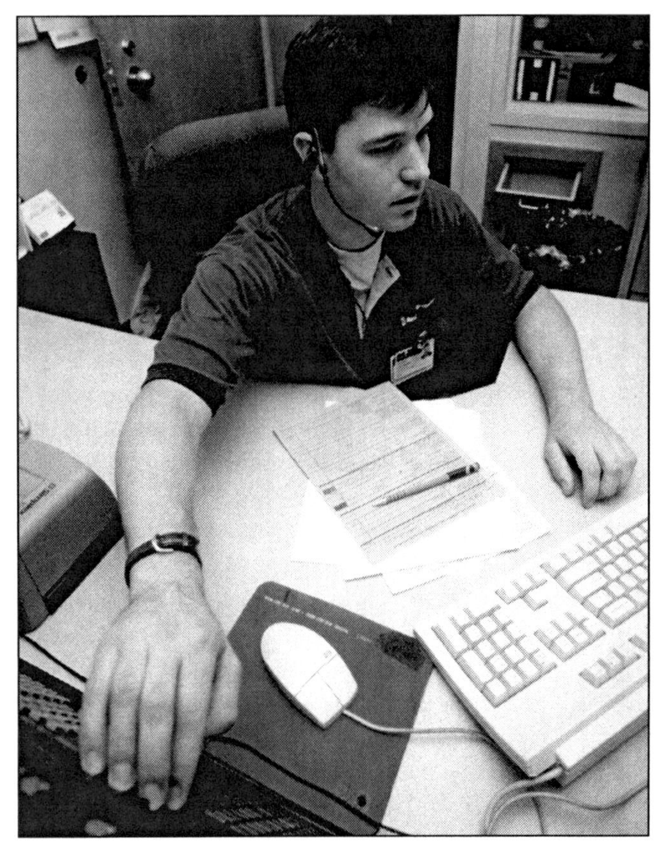

FIGURE 9-7 You will be assigned to a scene by the dispatcher.

The dispatcher should give the responding unit(s) the following information:

- The nature and severity of the injury, illness, or incident
- The exact location of the incident
- The number of patients
- Responses by other public safety agencies
- Special directions or advisories, such as adverse road or traffic conditions or severe weather reports
- The time at which the unit or units are dispatched

Your unit must confirm to the dispatcher that you have received the information and that you are en route to the scene. Local protocol will dictate whether it is the job of the dispatcher or your unit to notify other public safety agencies that you are responding to an emergency. In some areas, the emergency department is also notified whenever an ambulance responds to an emergency.

You should report any problems during your run to the dispatcher. You should also inform the dispatcher that you have arrived at the scene. The arrival report to the dispatcher should include any obvious details that you see during scene size up. For example, you might say, "Dispatcher, Medic One is on scene at Main Street with a two-vehicle collision."

All radio communications during dispatch, as well as other phases of operations, must be brief and easily understood. Although speaking in plain English is best, many areas find that 10 codes are shorter and simpler for routine communications. The development and use of such codes require strict discipline. When used improperly or not understood, codes create rather than clear up confusion.

Communicating with Medical Direction and Hospitals

The principal reason for radio communication is to facilitate communication between you and medical control (and the hospital). Medical control may be located at the receiving hospital, another facility, or sometimes even in another city or state. You must, however, consult with medical control to notify the hospital of an incoming patient, to request advice or orders from medical control, or to advise the hospital of special situations.

It is important to plan and organize your radio communication before you push the transmit button. *Remember, a concise, well-organized report demonstrates your competence and professionalism in the eyes of all who hear your report.* Well-organized radio communications with the hospital will engender confidence in the receiving facility's physicians and nurses, as well as others who are listening. In addition, the patient and family will be comforted by your organization and ability to communicate clearly. A well-delivered radio report puts you in control of the information-which is where you want to be.

Hospital notification is the most common type of communication between you and the hospital. The purpose of these calls is to notify the receiving facility of the patient's complaint and condition (Figure 9-8). On the basis of this information, the hospital is able to appropriately prepare staff and equipment to receive the patient.

Giving the patient report. The patient report should follow a standard format established by your EMS system. The patient report commonly includes the following seven elements:

1. **Your unit identification and level of services.** Example: "Brimfield Medical 71-BLS."
2. **The receiving hospital and your estimated time of arrival.** Example: "Robinson Memorial Hospital, ETA 10 minutes."
3. **The patient's age and gender.** Example: "A 33-year-old woman." The patient's name should not be given over the radio because it may be overheard. This is an invasion of the patient's privacy.
4. **The patient's chief complaint or your perception of the problem and its severity.** Example: "The patient complains of pain in the right lower leg."
5. **A brief history of the patient's current problem.** Example: "The patient fell down the steps." Other important history information that may pertain to the current problem should also be included, such as "The patient has diabetes and takes insulin."
6. **A brief report of physical findings.** This report should include level of consciousness, the patient's general appearance, pertinent abnormalities noted, and vital signs. Example: "The patient is alert and oriented and has normal color and warm skin. Her right lower leg is swollen and tender. Her blood pressure is 132 over 84, pulse is 72, and ventilations 14."
7. **A brief summary of the care given and any patient response.** Example: "We have immobilized the injured leg in a padded cardboard splint. The patient is now on a backboard. She still has motor, sensory, and circulatory function distal to the injured area. She also reports a decrease in pain since the splint was applied."

Be sure that you report all patient information in an objective, accurate, and professional manner. People with scanners are listening. You could be successfully sued for slander if you describe a patient in a way that injures his or her reputation.

The role of medical control. The delivery of EMS involves an impressive array of assessments, stabilization, and treatments. In some cases, you may assist patients in taking medications. Intermediate and advanced EMTs go beyond this level by initiating medication therapy based on the patient's presenting signs. For logical, ethical, and legal reasons, the delivery of such sophisticated care must be done in association with physicians. For this reason, every EMS system needs input and involvement from physicians. One or

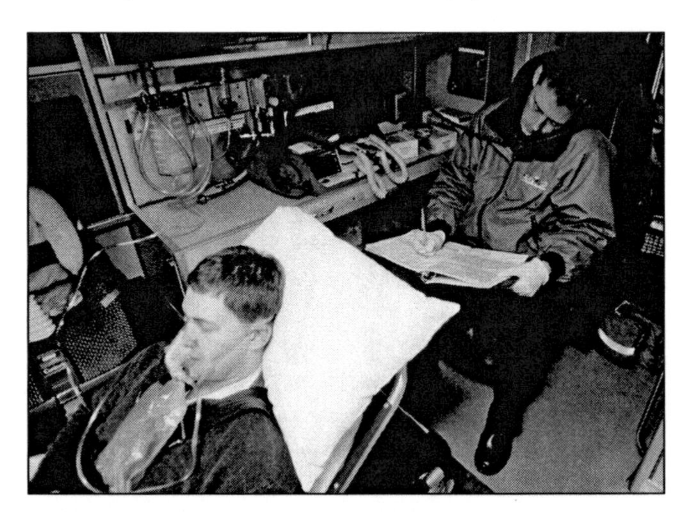

FIGURE 9-8 Giving the patient report should be done in an objective, accurate, professional manner.

more physicians, including your system or department medical director, will provide medical direction (medical control) for your EMS system. Medical control guides the treatment of patients in the system through protocols, direct orders and advice, and post-call review.

Depending upon how the protocols are written, you may need to call medical control for direct orders (permission) to administer certain treatments, to determine the transport destination of patients, or to be allowed to stop treatment and/or not transport a patient. In these cases, the radio or cellular phone provides a vital link between you and the expertise available through the base physician.

To maintain this link 24 hours a day, 7 days a week, medical control must be readily available on the radio at the hospital or on a mobile or portable unit when you call (Figure 9-9). In most areas, medical control is provided by the physicians who work at the receiving hospital. However, many variations have developed across the country. For example, some EMS units receive medical direction from one hospital even though they are taking the patient to another hospital. In other areas, medical direction may come from a free-standing center or even from an individual physician. Regardless of your system's design, your link to medical control is vital to maintain the high quality of care that your patient requires and deserves.

Calling medical control. You can use the radio in your unit or a portable radio to call medical control. A cellular telephone can also be used. Regardless of the type of radio, you should use a channel that is relatively free of other radio traffic and interference. There are a number of ways to control access on ambulance-to-hospital channels. In some EMS systems, the dispatcher monitors and assigns appropriate, clear medical control channels. Other EMS systems rely on special communications operations, such as CMEDs (Centralized Medical Emergency Dispatch) or resource coordination centers, to monitor and allocate the medical control channels.

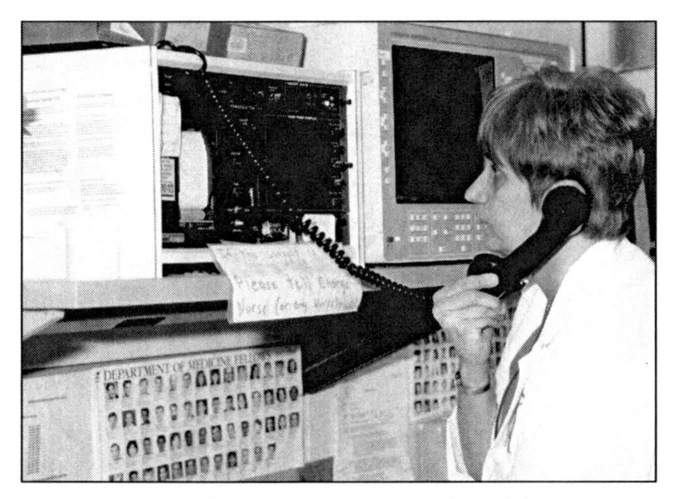

FIGURE 9-9 Medical control must be readily available on the radio at the hospital.

Because of the large number of EMS calls to medical control, your radio report must be well organized and precise and must contain only important information. In addition, because you need specific directions on patient care, the information that you provide to medical control must be accurate. *Remember, the physician on the other end bases his or her instructions on the information that you provide.*

You should never use codes when communicating with medical control unless you are directed by local protocol to do so. You should use proper medical terminology when giving your report. Never assume that medical control will know what a "10-50" or "Signal 70" means. Medical control handles many different EMS systems and will most likely not know your unit's special codes or signals.

To ensure complete understanding, once you receive an order from medical control, you must repeat the order back, word for word, and then receive confirmation. Whether the physician gives an order for medication or a specific treatment or denies a request for a particular treatment, you must repeat the order back word for word. This "echo" exchange helps to eliminate confusion and the possibility of poor patient care. *Orders that are unclear or seem inappropriate or incorrect should be questioned.* Do not blindly follow an order that does not make sense to you. The physician may have misunderstood or may have missed part of your report. In that case, he or she may not be able to respond appropriately to the patient's needs.

Information about special situations. Depending on your system's procedures, you may initiate communication with one or more hospitals to advise them of an extraordinary call or situation. For instance, a small rural hospital may be better able to respond to multiple victims of a highway crash if it is notified when the ambulance is first responding. At the other extreme, an entire hospital system must be notified of any disaster, such as a plane or train crash, as early as possible to enable activation of its staff call-in system. These special situations might also include HazMat situations, rescues in progress, multiple-casualty incidents, or any other situation that might require special preparation on the part of the hospital. In some areas, mutual aid frequencies may be designated in multiple-casualty incidents so that responding agencies can communicate with one another on a common frequency.

When notifying the hospital(s) of any special situations, keep the following in mind: The earlier the notification, the better. You should ask to speak to the charge nurse or physician in charge, as he or she is best able to mobilize the resources necessary to respond. Also, whenever possible, provide an estimate of the number of individuals who may be transported to the facility. Be sure to identify any special needs the patient(s) might have, such as burns or hazardous materials exposure, to assist the hospital in preparation. In many cases, hospital notification is part of a larger disaster or HazMat plan. Follow the plan for your system.

Standard Procedures and Protocols

You must use your radio communications system effectively from the time you acknowledge a call until you complete your run. Standard radio operating procedures are designed to reduce the number of misunderstood messages, to keep transmissions brief, and to develop effective radio discipline. Standard radio communications protocols help both you and the dispatcher to communicate properly (Table 9-1). Protocols should

TABLE 9-1 Guidelines for Effective Radio Communication

1. **Monitor the channel before transmitting** to avoid interfering with other radio traffic.
2. **Plan your message** before pushing the transmit switch. This will keep your transmissions brief and precise. You should use a standard format for your transmissions.
3. **Press the push-to-talk (PTT) button** on the radio, then wait for 1 second before starting your message. Otherwise, you might cut off the first part of your message before the transmitter is working at full power.
4. **Hold the microphone 2" to 3"** from your mouth. Speak clearly, but never shout into the microphone. Speak at a moderate, understandable rate, preferably in a clear, even voice.
5. **Identify the person or unit you are calling** first, then identify your unit as the sender. You will rarely work alone, so say "we" instead of "I" when describing yourself.
6. **Acknowledge a transmission** as soon as you can by saying, "Go ahead" or whatever is commonly used in your area. You should say, "Over and out," or whatever is commonly used in your area when you are finished. If you cannot take a long message, simply say, "Stand by" until you are ready.
7. **Use plain English.** Avoid meaningless phrases ("Be advised"), slang, or complex codes. Avoid words that are difficult to hear, such as "yes" and "no." Use "affirmative" and "negative."
8. **Keep your message brief.** If your message takes more than 30 seconds to send, pause after 30 seconds and say, "Do you copy?" The other party can then ask for clarification if needed. Also, someone else with emergency traffic can break through if necessary.
9. **Avoid voicing negative emotions,** such as anger or irritation, when transmitting. Courtesy is assumed, making it unnecessary to say "please" or "thank you," which wastes air time. Listen to other communications in your system to get a good idea of the common phrases and their uses.
10. **When transmitting a number** with two or more digits, say the entire number first and then each digit separately. For example, say, "sixty-seven," followed by "six-seven."
11. **Do not use profanity on the radio.** It is a violation of FCC rules and can result in substantial fines and even loss of your organization's radio license.
12. **Use EMS frequencies** for EMS communications. Do not use these frequencies for any other type of communications.
13. **Reduce background noise** as much as possible. Move away from wind, noisy motors, or tools. Close the window if you are in a moving ambulance. When possible, shut off the siren during radio transmissions.

include guidelines specifying a preferred format for transmitting messages, definitions of key words and phrases, and procedures for troubleshooting common radio communications problems.

The "call up" from one unit to another begins by identifying the called unit first, followed by the unit calling, such as "Dispatch, this is Medic One." This exchange alerts the dispatcher to listen for both the identity of the unit calling and the message.

Reporting Requirements

Proper use of the EMS communications system will help you to do your job more effectively. From acknowledgment of the call until you are cleared from the medical emergency, you will use radio communications. You must report in to dispatch at least six times during your run:

1. **To acknowledge the dispatch** information and to confirm that you are responding to the scene
2. **To announce your arrival** at the scene
3. **To announce that you are leaving** the scene and are en route to the receiving hospital. (At this point, you typically should also state the number of patients being transported, your estimated arrival time at the hospital, and the run status.)
4. **To announce your arrival** at the hospital or facility
5. **To announce that you are clear** of the incident or hospital and available for another assignment
6. **To announce your arrival** back at quarters or other off-the-air location

While en route to and from the scene, you should report to the dispatcher any special hazards or road conditions that might affect other responding units. Report any unusual delay, such as road blocks or elevated bridges. Once you are at the scene, you may request additional EMS or other public safety assistance and then help to coordinate their response.

During transport, you must periodically reassess the patient's overall condition, vital signs, and response to care provided. You should immediately report any significant changes in the patient's condition, especially if the patient seems worse. Medical control can then give new orders and prepare to receive the patient.

Maintenance of Radio Equipment

Like all other EMS equipment, radio equipment must be serviced by properly trained and equipped personnel. Remember that the radio is your lifeline to other public safety agencies (who function to protect you), as well as medical control, and it must perform under emergency conditions. Radio equipment that is operating properly should be serviced at least once a year. Any equipment that is not working properly should be immediately removed from service and sent for repair.

Sometimes, radio equipment will stop working during a run. In the worst-case scenario, it will stop just as you are trying to consult with medical control about treatment orders. Your EMS system must have several backup plans and options. The goal of a backup plan is to make sure that you can maintain contact with medical control when the usual procedures do not work. There are quite a few options.

The simplest backup plan relies on written standing orders. Standing orders are written documents that have been signed by the EMS system's medical director (Figure 9-10). These orders outline specific directions, permissions, and sometimes prohibitions regarding patient care. By their very nature, standing orders do not require direct communication with medical control. When properly followed, standing orders or formal protocols have the same authority and legal status as orders given over the radio. They exist to one extent or another in every EMS system and can be applied to all levels of EMS providers.

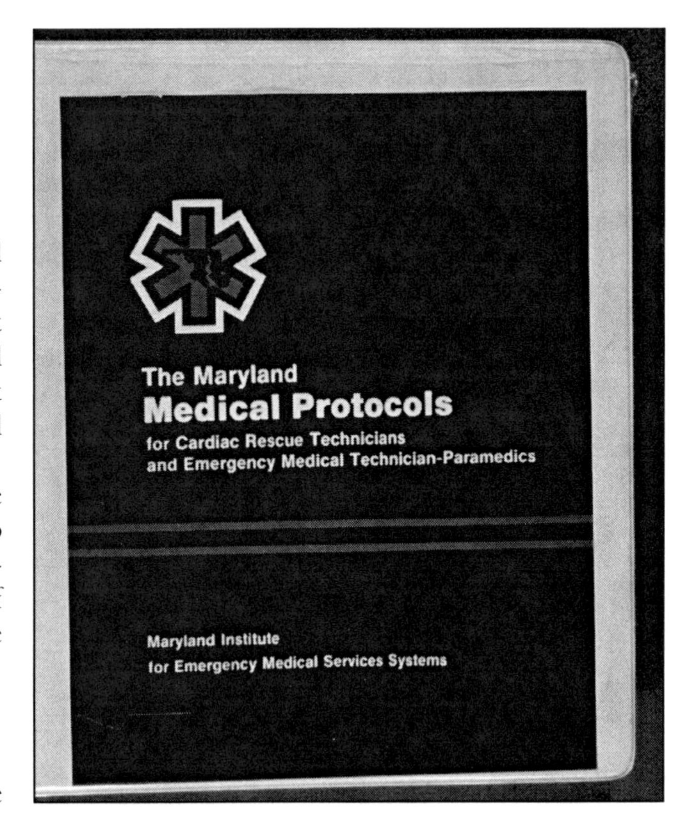

FIGURE 9-10 Standing orders are developed by the medical director and outline specific directions, permissions, and prohibitions regarding patient care.

Verbal Communications

As an EMT-B, you must master many communication skills, including radio operations and written communications. Verbal communications with the patient, the family, and the rest of the health care team are an essential part of high-quality patient care. And as an EMT-B, you must be able to find out what the patient needs and then tell others. *Never forget that you are the vital link between the patient and the remainder of the health care team.*

Communicating with Other Health Care Professionals

EMS is the first step in what is often a long and involved series of treatment phases. Effective communication between the EMT-B and health care professionals in the receiving facility is an essential cornerstone of efficient, effective, and appropriate patient care.

Your reporting responsibilities do not end when you arrive at the hospital. In fact, they have just begun. The transfer of care officially occurs during your oral report at the hospital, not as a result of your radio report en route. Once you arrive at the hospital, a hospital staff member will take responsibility of the patient from you (Figure 9-11). Depending on the hospital and the condition of the patient, the training of the person who takes over the care of the patient varies. However, you may transfer the care of your patient only to someone with at least your level of training. Once a hospital staff member is ready to take responsibility for the patient, you must provide that person with a formal oral report of the patient's condition.

Giving a report is a longstanding and well-documented part of transferring the patient's care from one provider to another. Your oral report is usually given at the same time that the staff member is doing something for the patient. For example, a nurse or physician may be looking at the patient, beginning assessment, or helping you to move the patient from the stretcher to an examination table. Therefore, you must report important information in a complete, precise way. The following six components must be included in the oral report:

1. **The patient's name** (if you know it) and the chief complaint, nature of illness, or mechanism of injury. Example: "This is Mr. Campbell. His wife told us that he has been acting confused all day."
2. **A summary of the information** that you gave in your radio report. Example: "He has a history of high blood pressure and had a stroke 4 years ago. He has little permanent damage from the stroke. His wife states that he is usually alert and oriented."
3. **Any important history** that was not given already. Example: "His wife told us that he takes his medicine regularly. On the way in, she told us that Mr. Campbell's medicine was just changed 2 days ago."
4. **The patient's response to treatment** given en route. It is especially important to report any changes in the patient or the treatment provided since your radio report. Example: "We started oxygen by face mask at 10 L/min. His LOC improved, and he started to fight the mask. We were able to get him to hold the mask next to his mouth and nose for the rest of the trip."
5. **The vital signs assessed** during transport and after the radio report. Example: "His vitals during transport were blood pressure 184 over 110, pulse 96, ventilations 22. They are generally unchanged since we reported earlier."
6. **Any other information** that you may have gathered that was not important enough to report sooner. Information that was gathered during transport, any patient medications you have brought with you, and any other details about the patient that was provided by family members or friends may be included. Example: "Mrs. Jones's husband rode in with us. Her daughter is coming from home and should be here soon."

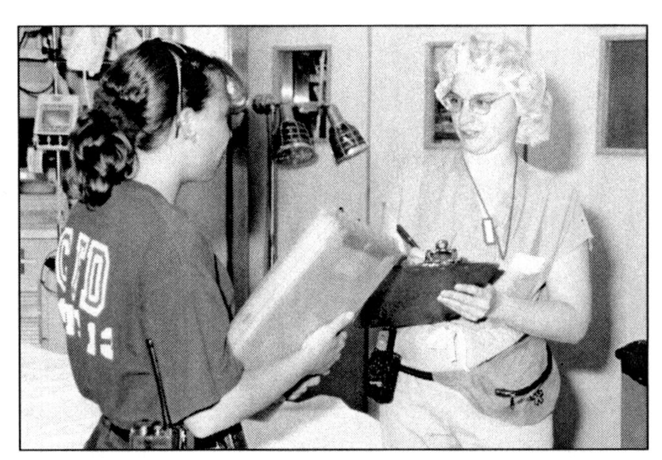

FIGURE 9-11 Once you arrive at the hospital, a staff member will take responsibility for the patient from you.

Communicating with Patients

Your communication skills will be tested when you communicate with patients and/or families. Remember that someone who is sick or injured is scared and might not understand what you are doing and saying. Therefore, your gestures, body movements, and attitude toward the patient are critically important in gaining the trust of both patient and family. These *Ten Golden Rules* will help you to calm and reassure your patients:

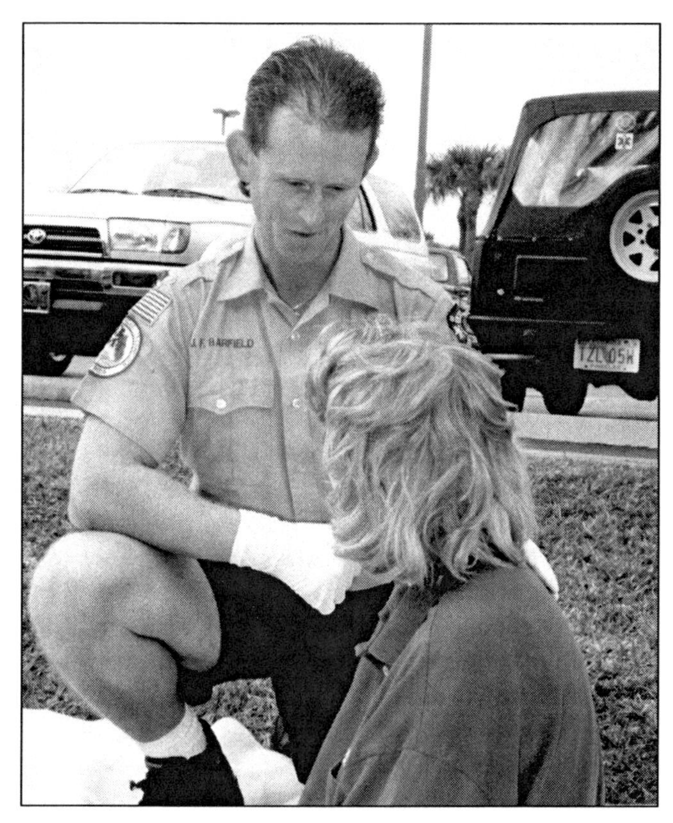

FIGURE 9-12 Maintaining eye contact with your patient builds trust and lets patient know that he or she is your first priority.

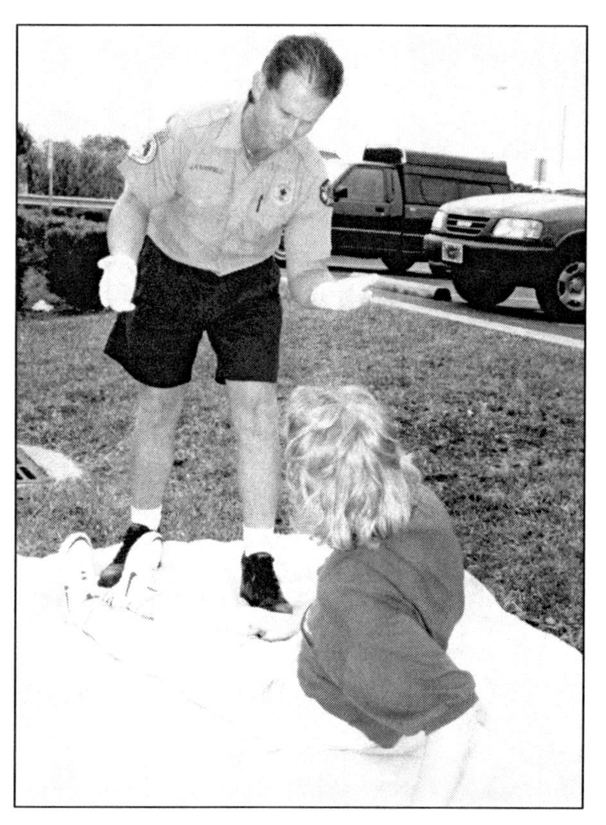

FIGURE 9-13 Watch your body language, as patients may misinterpret your gestures, movements, and stance.

1. **Make and keep eye contact** with your patient at all times (Figure 9-12). Give the patient your undivided attention. This will let the patient know that he or she is your top priority. Look the patient straight in the eye to establish rapport. Establishing rapport is building a trusting relationship with your patient. This will make the job of caring for the patient much easier for both you and the patient.
2. **Use the patient's proper name** when you know it. Ask the patient what he or she wishes to be called. Do not use terms such as "Pops," "Lady," "Kid," or "Dear." Avoid using a patient's first name unless the patient is a child or the patient asks you to use his or her first name. Rather, use a courtesy title, such as "Mr. Peters," "Mrs. Smith," or "Ms. Butler."
3. **Tell the patient the truth.** Even if you have to say something very unpleasant, telling the truth is better than lying. Lying will destroy the patient's trust in you and decrease your own confidence. You might not always tell the patient everything, but if the patient or a family member asks a specific question, you should answer truthfully. A direct question deserves a direct answer. If you do not know the answer to the patient's question, say so. For example, a patient may ask, "Am I having a heart attack?" "I don't know" is an adequate answer.
4. **Use language that the patient can understand.** Do not talk up or down to the patient in any way. Avoid technical medical terms that the patient might not understand. For example, ask the patient whether he or she has a history of "heart problems." This will usually result in more accurate information than if you ask about "previous episodes of myocardial infarction" or a "history of cardiomyopathy."
5. **Be careful of what you say** about the patient to others. A patient might hear only part of what is said. As a result, the patient might seriously misinterpret (and remember for a long time) what was said. Therefore, assume that the patient can hear every word you say, even if you are speaking to others and even if the patient appears to be unconscious or unresponsive.
6. **Be aware of your body language** (Figure 9-13). Nonverbal communication is extremely important in dealing with patients. In stressful situations, patients may misinterpret your gestures and movements. Be particularly careful not to appear threatening. Instead, position yourself at a lower level than the patient when practical. Remember that you should always, always conduct yourself in a calm, professional manner.

7. **Always speak slowly,** clearly, and distinctly.
8. **If the patient is hearing impaired,** speak clearly, and face the person so that he or she can read your lips. Do not shout at a person who is hearing impaired. Shouting will not make it any easier for the patient to understand you. Instead, it may frighten the patient and make it even more difficult for the patient to understand you. Never assume that an elderly patient is hearing impaired or otherwise unable to understand you. Also, never use baby talk with elderly patients or with anyone but babies.
9. **Allow time for the patient to answer** or respond to your questions. Do not rush a patient unless there is immediate danger. Sick and injured people may not be thinking clearly and may need time to answer even simple questions. This is especially true in treating elderly patients.
10. **Act and speak in a calm, confident manner** while caring for the patient. Make sure that you attend to the patient's pains and needs. Try to make the patient physically comfortable and relaxed. Find out whether the patient is more comfortable sitting or lying down. Is the patient cold or hot? Does the patient want a friend or relative nearby?

Patients literally place their lives in your hands. They deserve to know that you can provide medical care and that you are concerned about their well-being.

Patients deserve to know that you can provide medical care and that you are concerned about their well-being.

Communicating with Elderly Patients

By the year 2000, about 13% of the U.S. population will be considered geriatric, or over age 65 years. A person's actual age might not be the most important factor in making him or her "elderly." It is more important to determine a person's functional age. The functional age relates to the person's ability to function in daily activities, the person's mental state, and activity pattern.

Most elderly people think clearly, can give you a clear medical history, and can answer your questions (Figure 9-14). *Do not assume that an elderly patient is senile or confused.* Remember, though, that communicating with some elderly patients is extremely difficult. Some may be hostile, irritable, and/or confused. Others may have difficulty hearing or seeing you. You need great patience and compassion when you are called upon to care for such a patient. Think of the patient as someone's grandmother or grandfather—or even as yourself when you reach that age.

Approach an elderly patient slowly and calmly. Allow plenty of time for the patient to respond to your questions. Watch for signs of confusion, anxiety, or impaired hearing or vision. The patient should feel confident that you are in charge and that everything possible is being done for him or her.

Elderly patients often do not feel much pain. An elderly person who has fallen or been injured may report no pain. In addition, elderly patients might not be fully aware of important changes in other body systems. As a result, be especially vigilant for objective changes—no matter how subtle-in their condition. Even minor changes in breathing or mental state may signal major problems.

Remember to attend to an elderly patient's family members and friends. Seeing a loved one taken away in an ambulance can be a particularly frightening experience. Take a few minutes to explain to an elderly patient's spouse or family what is being done and why such action is being taken. When possible (which is more often than you'd think), give the patient some time to pack a few personal items before leaving for the hospital. Be sure to get any hearing aids, glasses, or dentures packed before departure; it will make the patient's hospital stay much more pleasant. You might want to document on the prehospital care report that these items accompanied the patient to the hospital and were given to a specific staff person in the emergency department.

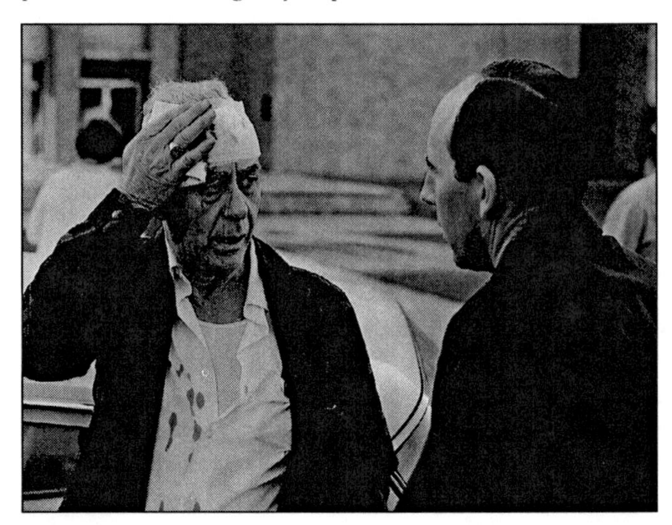

FIGURE 9-14 You need a great deal of compassion and patience when caring for the elderly, but do not assume that the patient is senile or confused.

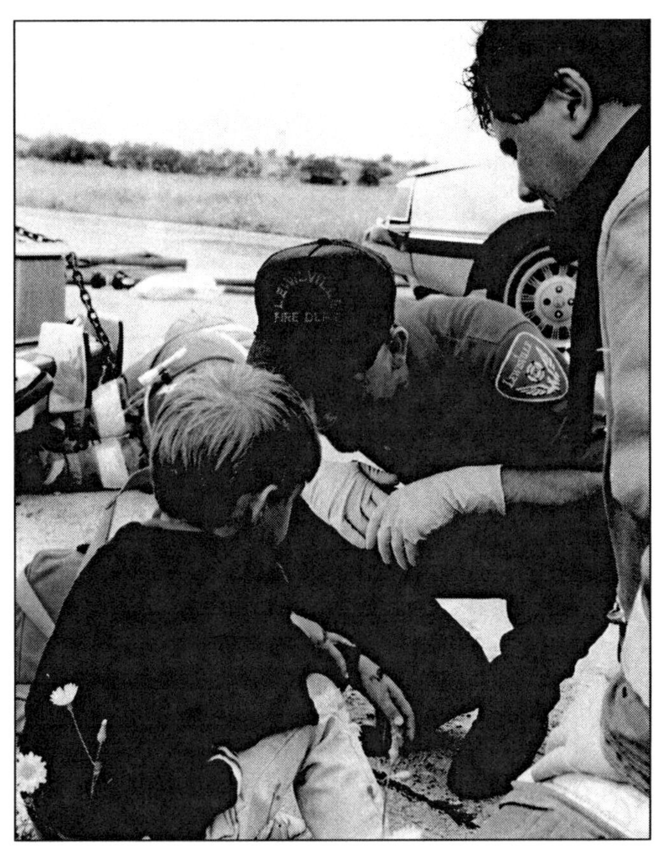

FIGURE 9-15 Maintain eye contact with a child to let the child know that you are there to help and that you can be trusted.

Communicating with Children

Everyone who is thrust into an emergency situation becomes frightened to some degree. However, fear is probably most severe and most obvious in children. Children may be frightened by your uniform, the ambulance, and the number of people who have suddenly gathered around. Even a child who says little may be very much aware of all that is going on.

Familiar objects and faces will help to reduce this fright. Let a child keep a favorite toy, doll, or security blanket to give the child some sense of control and comfort. Having a family member or friend nearby is also helpful. When not contraindicated by the child's condition, it is often helpful to let the parent or an adult friend hold the child during your evaluation and treatment. However, you will have to make sure that this person will not upset the child. Sometimes, adult family members are not helpful because they become too upset by what has happened. An overly anxious parent or relative can make things worse. Be careful about selecting the proper adult for this role.

Children can easily see through lies or deceptions, so you must always be honest with them. Make sure that you explain to the child over and over again what and why certain things are happening. If treatment is going to hurt, such as applying a splint, tell the child ahead of time. Also tell the child that it will not hurt for long and that it will help "make it better."

Respect a child's modesty. Both little girls and little boys are often embarrassed if they have to undress or be undressed in front of strangers. This phobia further intensifies during adolescence. When a wound or site of injury has to be exposed, try to do so out of sight of strangers. Again, it is extremely important to tell the child what you are doing and why you are doing it.

You should speak to a child in a professional yet friendly way. A child should feel reassured that you are there to help in every way possible. Maintain eye contact with a child, as you would with an adult, to let the child know that you are helping and that you can be trusted (Figure 9-15). It is helpful to position yourself at their level so that you do not appear to tower above them.

Communicating with Hearing-Impaired Patients

Patients who are hearing impaired or deaf are usually not ashamed or embarrassed by their disability. Often, it is the people around a deaf or hearing-impaired person who have the problem coping. Remember that you must be able to communicate with hearing-impaired patients so that you can provide necessary or even lifesaving care.

First, you should always assume that hearing-impaired patients have normal intelligence. These patients can usually understand what is going on around them, provided that you can successfully communicate with them. Second, most patients who are hearing impaired can read lips to some extent. Therefore, you should place yourself in a position so that the patient can see your lips. Third, many hearing-impaired patients have hearing aids that may have been lost in an accident or fall. Hearing aids may also be forgotten if the patient is confused or ill. Look around, or ask the patient or the family about a hearing aid.

Remember the following five steps to help you efficiently communicate with patients who are hearing impaired:

1. **Have paper and a pen available.** This way, you can write down questions and the patient can write down answers if necessary. Be sure to print so that your handwriting is not a communications barrier.
2. **If the patient can read lips,** you should face the patient and speak slowly and distinctly. Do not cover your mouth or mumble. If it is night or dark, consider shining a light on your face.

3. **Never shout!**
4. **Be sure to listen carefully,** ask short questions, and give short answers. Remember that although many hearing-impaired patients can speak distinctly, some cannot.
5. **Learn some simple phrases** in sign language. For example, knowing the signs for "sick," "hurt," and "help" may be useful if you cannot communicate in any other way (Figure 9-16).

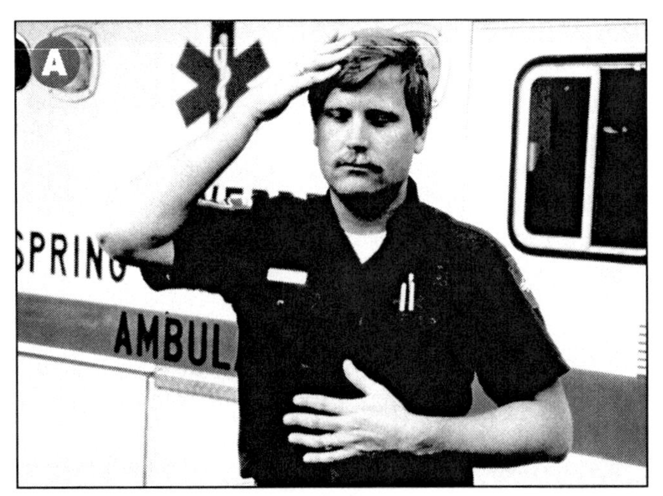

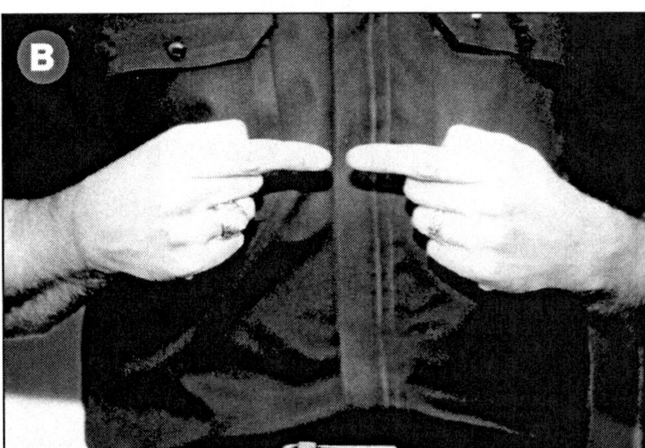

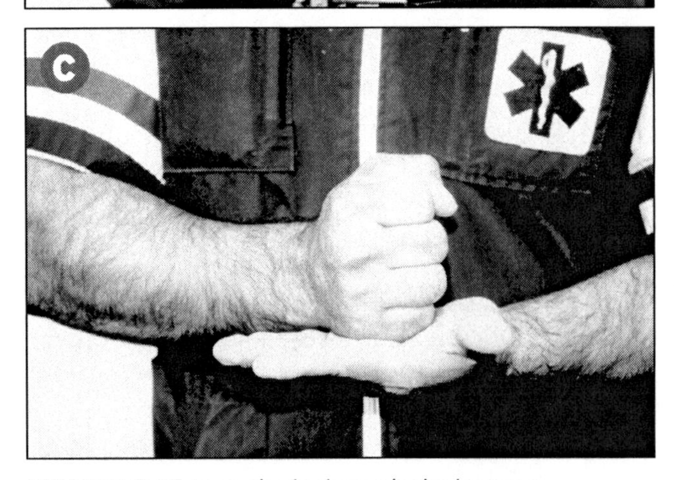

FIGURE 9-16 Learn simple phrases in sign language.
A: Sick. **B:** Hurt. **C:** Help.

Communicating with Visually Impaired Patients

Like hearing-impaired patients, visually impaired and blind patients have usually accepted and learned to deal with their disability. Of course, not all visually impaired patients are completely blind. Many can perceive light and dark or can see shadows or movement. Ask the patient whether he or she can see at all. Also remember that, as with other patients who have disabilities, you should expect that visually impaired patients have normal intelligence.

As you begin caring for a visually impaired patient, explain everything that you are doing in detail as you are doing it. Be sure to stay in physical contact with the patient as you begin your care. Hold your hand lightly on the patient's shoulder or arm. Try to avoid sudden movements. If the patient can walk to the ambulance, place his or her hand on your arm, taking care not to rush. Transport any mobility aids, such as a cane, with the patient to the hospital. A visually impaired person may have a guide dog. Guide dogs are easily identified by their special harnesses. They are trained not to leave their masters and not to respond to strangers (Figure 9-17). A visually impaired patient who is conscious can tell you

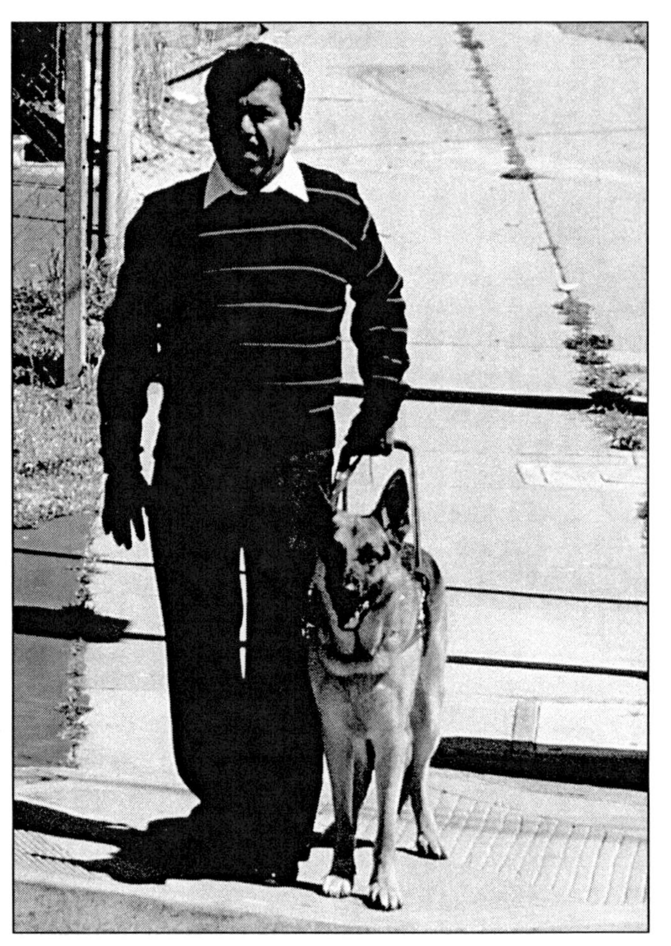

FIGURE 9-17 A guide dog is easily identified by its special harness.

about the dog and give instructions for its care. If circumstances permit, bring the guide dog to the hospital with the patient. If the dog has to be left behind, you should arrange for its care.

Communicating with Non-English-Speaking Patients

As part of the focused physical exam, you must obtain a medical history from the patient. You cannot skip this step simply because the patient does not speak English. Most patients who do not speak English fluently will still know certain important words or phrases.

Your first step is to find out how much English the patient can speak. Use short, simple questions and simple words whenever possible. Avoid difficult medical terms. You can help patients to better understand if you point to specific parts of the body as you ask questions.

In many areas, particularly large urban centers, major segments of the population do not speak English. Your job will be much easier if you learn some common words and phrases in their language, especially common medical terms. Pocket cards are available that show the pronunciation of these terms. If the patient does not speak any English, find a family member or friend to act as an interpreter.

Written Communications and Documentation

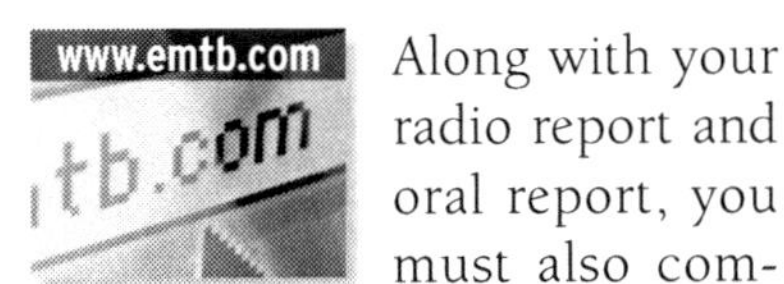

Along with your radio report and oral report, you must also complete a formal written report about the patient before you leave the hospital. You might be able to do the written report en route, if the trip is long enough and the patient needs minimal care. Usually, you will finish the written report after you have transferred the care of the patient to a hospital staff member. Be sure to leave the report at the hospital before you leave.

Minimum Data Set

The information that you collect during a call becomes part of the data set. The minimum data set includes both patient information and administrative information (Figure 9-18). The patient information that is included in the minimum data set should be as follows:

- Chief complaint
- Level of consciousness (AVPU) or mental status

PRESS FIRMLY — USE BALLPOINT PEN — YOU ARE WRITING ON A 5 PAGE FORM

NORTH AMERICAN PRESS, INC. (708) 483-1400

Good Samaritan
EMS System Ambulance Report

Serial # 49305 — Incident # 256785 — Patient 1 of 1

Department ROSEMONT FIRE DEPT. — Department # 12 — License 73267 — Unit # 155 — Date 07/04/95 — Service Provided ALS / BLS / REF

LOCATION: 1623 MAIN ST.

PATIENT INFORMATION NAME (Last) JONES (First) JANET

ADDRESS 1623 MAIN ST APT 623

CITY ROSEMONT STATE IL ZIP 60018

AGE 65 D.O.B. 07/03/30 SEX F WEIGHT 120 PHONE 708-123-4567

INITIAL IMPRESSION: ULCER COMPLICATIONS

CHIEF COMPLAINT: ABDOMINAL PAIN

MEDICATIONS ☐ Denies: TAGAMET, LOPRESSOR

MEDICAL HISTORY ☐ Denies ☒ HTN ☐ Cardiac ☐ Diabetes ☐ COPD ☐ Seizures ☐ Cancer — PEPTIC ULCERS — Last Menstrual Period

ALLERGIES ☒ Denies ☐ PCN ☐ Codeine ☐ Sulfa ☐ Iodine

Times: 0830 Call Rec'd; 0830 Responding; 0834 Arrived Scene; 0908 Enroute Hosp.; 0920 Arrived Hosp.; 0950 Depart Hosp; 0959 Back in Service

CREW # / NAME: A) 1457; B) TURNER 1437; C); D); E) — ☐ Gloves ☐ Gown ☐ Mask ☐ Eyeshield

BODY FLUID EXPOSURE ☐ A ☐ B ☐ C ☐ D ☐ E

MEDICAL CONTROL HOSP. GENERAL

RADIO LOG # 16275

HOSP. TRANSPORTED TO RESURRECTION MC

TRAFFIC DELAYED BY TRAIN ☐ Light ☒ Medium ☐ Heavy ☐ Clear ☒ Wet ☐ Snow ☐ Ice

INITIAL: TIME 0837 — EYES 4 Spont — VERBAL 5 Orient — MOTOR 6 Obeys — GCS 15 — SKIN COLOR ☒ Pale/Ashen — TEMP. ☒ Normal — MOISTURE ☒ Normal — PUPILS ☒ PERL — LUNGS ☒ Clear — ☒ Blood Sugar 100 — FIELD TRAUMA SCORE

TIME	NEURO	B/P	PULSE	RESPS	TIME	ECG RHYTHM / DEFIB	TIME	DRUG / SOLUTION	DOSE	ROUTE
0839	(A)VPU	110/78	82 SR	16 NR	0840	NSR	0845	.9% SALINE	1000 cc	IV
0855	(A)VPU	118/76	84 SR	16 NR	0855	NSR				
	AVPU									
	AVPU									
	AVPU									

FINAL: TIME 0919 — EYES 4 Spont — VERBAL 5 Orient — MOTOR 6 Obeys — GCS 15 — SKIN COLOR ☒ Normal — TEMP. ☒ Normal — MOISTURE ☒ Normal — PUPILS ☒ PERL — LUNGS ☒ Clear — FIELD TRAUMA SCORE

COMMENTS / FINDINGS: PATIENT COMPLAINED OF EPIGASTRIC PAIN. PATIENT STATES SHE HAS BEEN UNDER STRESS AND HAS NOT TAKEN HER MEDICATION. PT DENIES CHEST PAIN. PT STATES NORMAL BOWEL MOVEMENTS. PT COMPLAINS OF NAUSEA BUT DENIES VOMITING

PROCEDURES (A B C D E): Airway - Manual; Airway - OP/NP; Airway - OT/NT; Airway Unable; Assessment; Communication; Cricothyroidotomy; Defib/Cardioversion; ECG Interpretation; IV/IO Start; IV/IO Unable; Medications Admin; OB Delivery; Pacemaker; Pleural Decomp; Restraints; Spine Immob; Splint Limb; Other; Other

☐ Continuation sheet

PROVIDER AGENCY

FIGURE 9-18 The minimum data set includes both patient information and administrative information.

- Systolic blood pressure for patients older than age 3 years
- Capillary refill for patients younger than age 6 years
- Skin color and temperature
- Pulse
- Respirations and effort

The administrative information that is included in the minimum data set should be as follows:

- The time that the incident was reported
- The time that the EMS unit was notified
- The time that the EMS unit arrived at the scene
- The time that the EMS unit left the scene
- The time that the EMS unit arrived at the receiving facility
- The time that patient care was transferred

You will begin gathering the patient information as soon as you reach the patient. Continue collecting information as you provide care until you arrive at the hospital.

Prehospital Care Report

Prehospital care reports help to ensure efficient continuity of patient care. This report describes the nature of the patient's injuries or illness at the scene and the initial treatment you provide. Although this report might not be read immediately at the hospital, it may very well be referred to later for important information. The prehospital care report serves the following six functions:

1. Continuity of care
2. Legal documentation
3. Education
4. Administrative
5. Research
6. Evaluation and continuous quality improvement

A good prehospital care report documents the care that was provided and the patient's condition on arrival at the scene. It also documents any changes in the patient's condition upon arrival at the hospital. The information in the report also proves that you have provided proper documentation. In some instances, it also shows that you have properly handled unusual or uncommon situations. Both objective and subjective information is included in this report. *It is critical that you document everything in the clearest manner possible.* If a patient brings legal action against you, you and your prehospital care report will have to go to court.

These reports also provide valuable administrative information. For example, the report provides information for patient billing. It can also be used to evaluate response times, equipment usage, and other areas of administrative responsibility.

Data may be obtained from the prehospital care forms to analyze causes, severity, and types of illness or injury requiring emergency medical care. These reports may also be used in an ongoing program for evaluation of the quality of patient care. All records are reviewed periodically by your system. The purpose of this review is to make sure that trauma triage and/or other prehospital care criteria have been met.

There are many requirements on a prehospital care report (Table 9-2). Often, these requirements vary from jurisdiction to jurisdiction, mainly because so many agencies obtain information from them. There is no universally accepted form.

Types of Forms

You will most likely use one of two types of forms. The first type is the traditional written form with check boxes and a narrative section. The second type is a computerized version in which you fill in information using an electronic clipboard or similar device (Figure 9-19). If your service uses written forms, be sure to fill in the boxes completely, and avoid making stray marks on the sheet. Make sure that you are familiar with the specific procedures for collecting, recording, and reporting the information in your area.

If you must complete a narrative section, be sure to describe what you see and what you do. Be sure to include significant negative findings and important observations about the scene. Do not record your conclusions about the incident. For example, you may write, "The patient's breath smelled of alcohol." This is a clear description that does not make any judgments about the patient's condition. However, a report that says, "The patient was drunk," makes a conclusion about the patient's condition. Also avoid radio codes, and use only standard abbreviations. When information is of a sensitive nature, note the source of the information. Be sure to spell words correctly, especially medical terms. If you do not know how to spell a particular word, find out how to spell it, or use another word. Also be sure to record the time with all assessment findings.

TABLE 9-2 Components of Prehospital Care Report

- Patient's name, gender, date of birth, and address
- Nature of the call
- Mechanism of injury
- Location of the patient when first seen (including specific details, especially if the incident is a car accident or criminal activity is suspected)
- Rescue and treatment given before your arrival
- Signs and symptoms found during your patient assessment
- Care and treatment given at the site and during transport
- Baseline vital signs
- SAMPLE history changes in vital signs and condition
- Date of the call
- Time of the call
- Location of the call
- Time of dispatch
- Time of arrival at the scene
- Time of leaving the scene
- Time of arrival at the hospital
- Patient's insurance information
- Names and/or certification numbers of the EMT-Bs who responded to the call
- Name of the base hospital involved in the run
- Type of run to the scene: emergency or routine

Falsifying information on the prehospital report may result in suspension and/or revocation of your certification/license.

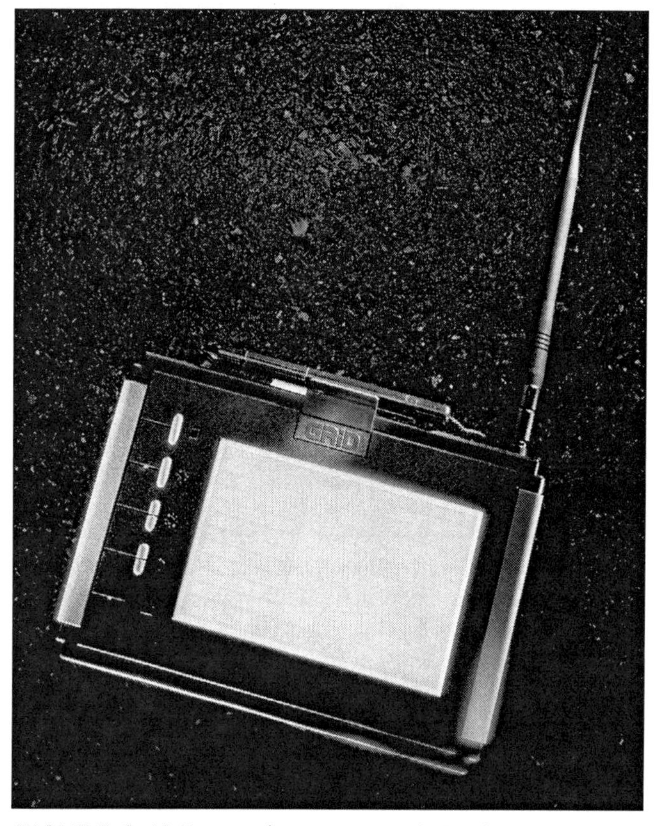

FIGURE 9-19 Your service may use an electronic clipboard, which is a computerized version of the traditional written form.

Remember that the report form itself and all the information on it are considered confidential documents. Be sure that you are familiar with state and local laws concerning confidentiality. All prehospital forms must be handled with care and stored in an appropriate manner once you have completed them. After you have completed a report, distribute the copies to the appropriate locations, according to state and local protocol. In most instances, a copy of the report will remain at the hospital and will become a part of the patient's record.

Reporting Errors

Everyone makes mistakes. If you leave something out of a report or record information incorrectly, do not try to cover it up. Rather, write down what did or did not happen and the steps that were taken to correct the situation. Falsifying information on the prehospital report may result in suspension and/or revocation of your certification/license. More important, falsifying information results in poor patient care, because other health care providers have a false impression of assessment findings or the treatment given. Document only

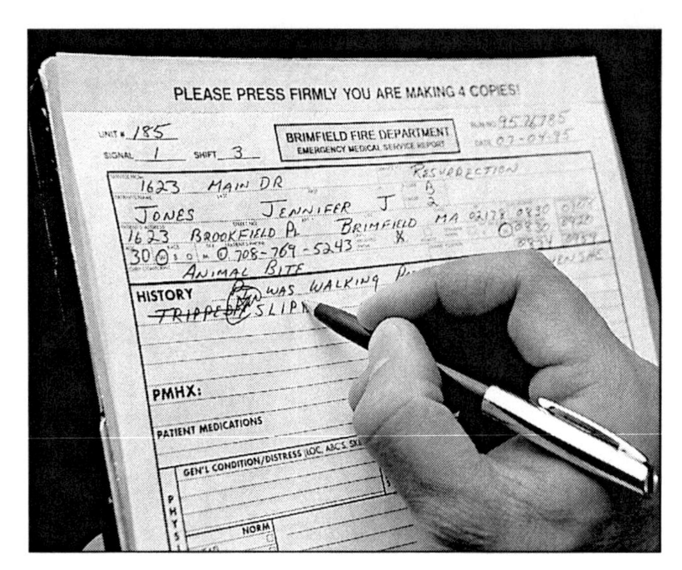

FIGURE 9-20 If you make a mistake in writing your report, the proper way to correct it is to draw a single horizontal line through the error, initial it, and write the correct information next to it.

the vital signs that were actually taken. If you did not give the patient oxygen, do not chart that the patient was given oxygen.

If you discover an error as you are writing your report, draw a single horizontal line through the error, initial it, and write the correct information next to it (Figure 9-20). Do not try to erase or cover the error with correction fluid. This may be interpreted as an attempt to cover up a mistake.

If an error is discovered after you submit your report, draw a single line through the error, preferably in a different color ink, initial it, and date it. Make sure to add a note with the correct information. If you left out information accidentally, add a note with the correct information, the date, and your initials.

When you do not have enough time to complete your report before the next call, you will need to fill it out later.

Usually, you will finish the written report after you have transferred the care of the patient to a hospital staff member. Be sure to leave the report at the hospital before you leave.

Documenting Right of Refusal

Competent adult patients have the right to refuse treatment (Figure 9-21). If you are faced with this situation, you must inform medical control immediately. Before you leave the scene, try to persuade the patient to go to the hospital, and consult medical direction as directed by local protocol. Also make sure that the patient is able to make a rational, informed decision and is not under the influence of alcohol or other drugs or the effects of an illness or injury. Explain to the patient why it is important to be examined by a physician at the hospital. Also explain what may happen if the patient is not examined by a physician. If the patient still refuses, suggest other means for the patient to obtain proper care. Explain that you are willing to return. If the patient still refuses, document any assessment findings and emergency medical care given, then have the patient sign a refusal form. You must also have a family member, police officer, or bystander sign the form as a witness. If the patient refuses to sign the refusal form, have a family member, police officer, or bystander sign the form verifying that the patient refused to sign.

Be sure to complete the prehospital report, including the patient assessment findings. Also include a description of the care that you wished to provide for the patient. You must also include a statement explaining that you informed the patient of the possible consequences of failure to accept care, including potential death, and alternative methods of obtaining the care that you suggested.

Special Reporting Situations

In some instances, you may be required to file special reports with appropriate authorities. These may include incidents involving gunshot wounds, dog bites, certain infectious diseases, or suspected physical, sexual, or substance abuse. Learn your local requirements for reporting these incidents. Failure to report them may have legal consequences. It is important that the report be accurate, objective, and submitted in a timely manner. Also remember to keep a copy for your own records.

Another special reporting situation is a multiple-casualty incident (MCI). The local MCI plan should have some means of recording important medical information temporarily (such as a triage tag that can be used later to complete the form). The standard for completing the form in an MCI is not the same as for a typical call. Your local plan should have specific guidelines.

RELEASE FROM RESPONSIBILITY WHEN PATIENT REFUSES IV THERAPY

This is to certify that I, ______________________________ (patient's name), am refusing IV treatment. I acknowledge that I have been informed of the risk involved and hereby release the emergency medical services provider(s), the physician consultant, and the consulting hospital from all responsibility for any ill effects which may result from this action.

Witness ______________________________ Signed ______________________________ (patient name or nearest relative)

Witness ______________________________ ______________________________ (relationship)

RELEASE FROM RESPONSIBILITY WHEN PATIENT REFUSES SERVICE

This is to certify that I, ______________________________ (patient's name), am refusing the services offered by the emergency medical services provider(s). I acknowledge that I have been informed of the risk involved and hereby release the emergency medical services provider(s), the physician consultant, and the consulting hospital from all responsibility for any ill effects which may result from this action.

Witness ______________________________ Signed ______________________________ (patient name or nearest relative)

Witness ______________________________ ______________________________ (relationship)

RELEASE FROM RESPONSIBILITY WHEN PATIENT REFUSES SERVICES BUT ACCEPTS TRANSPORT

This is to certify that I, ______________________________ (patient's name), am refusing ______________________________ ______________________________. I acknowledge that I have been informed of the risk involved and hereby release the emergency medical services provider(s), the physician consultant, and the consulting hospital from all responsibility for any ill effects which may result from this action. However, I do accept transportation to a medical facility.

Witness ______________________________ Signed ______________________________ (patient name or nearest relative)

Witness ______________________________ ______________________________ (relationship)

FIGURE 9-21 A competent adult patient has the right to refuse medical treatment and must sign a refusal form.

prep kit

ready for review

Excellent communication skills are crucial in relaying pertinent information to the hospital before arrival. Radio and telephone communication links you and your team to other members of the EMS, fire, and law enforcement communities. This enables your entire team to work together more effectively. It is your job to know what your communication system can and cannot handle. You must be able to communicate effectively by sending precise, accurate reports about the scene, the patient's condition, and the treatment that you provide.

There are many different forms of communication that an EMT-B must understand and be able to use. First, you must be familiar with two-way radio communications and have a working knowledge of mobile and hand-held portable radios. You must know when to use them and what type of information you can transmit. Remember, the lines of communication are not always exclusive; therefore, you should speak in a professional manner at all times.

In addition to radio and oral communications with hospital personnel, EMT-B's must have excellent person-to-person communication skills. You should be able to interact with the patient and any family members, friends, or bystanders. It is important for you to remember that people who are sick or injured may not understand what you are doing or saying. Therefore, your body language and attitude are very important in gaining the trust of both the patient and family. You must also take special care of individuals such as children, the elderly, and hearing-impaired, visually impaired, and non-English-speaking patients.

Along with your radio report and oral report, you must also complete a formal written report about the patient before you leave the hospital. This is a vital part of providing emergency medical care and ensuring the continuity of patient care. This information guarantees the proper transfer of responsibility, complies with the requirements of health departments and law enforcement agencies, and fulfills your administrative needs. Reporting and record-keeping duties are essential, but they should never come before the care of a patient.

vital vocabulary

www.emtb.com

base station Any radio hardware containing a transmitter and receiver that is located in a fixed place.

cellular telephone A low-power portable radio that communicates through an interconnected series of repeater stations called "cells."

channel An assigned frequency or frequencies that are used to carry voice and/or data communications.

dedicated line A special telephone line that is used for specific point-to-point communications; also known as a "hot line."

duplex The ability to transmit and receive simultaneously.

Federal Communications Commission (FCC) The federal agency that has jurisdiction over interstate and international telephone and telegraph services and satellite communications, all of which may involve EMS activity.

MED channels VHF and UHF channels that the FCC has designated exclusively for EMS use.

paging The use of a radio signal and a voice or digital message that is transmitted to pagers ("beepers") or desktop monitor radios.

rapport A trusting relationship that you build with your patient.

repeater A special base station radio that receives messages and signals on one frequency and then automatically retransmits them on a second frequency.

scanner A radio receiver that searches or "scans" across several frequencies until the message is completed; the process is then repeated.

simplex Single-frequency radio; transmissions can occur in either direction but not simultaneously in both; when one party transmits, the other can only receive, and the party that is transmitting is unable to receive.

standing orders Written documents, signed by the EMS system's medical director, that outline specific directions, permissions, and sometimes prohibitions regarding patient care; also called protocols.

telemetry A process in which electronic signals are converted into coded, audible signals; these signals can then be transmitted by radio or telephone to a receiver at the hospital with a decoder.

UHF (ultra-high frequency) Radio frequencies between 300 and 3,000 MHz.

VHF (very high frequency) Radio frequencies between 30 and 300 MHz; the VHF spectrum is further divided into "high" and "low" bands.

assessment in action

You are transporting a patient from an extended care facility to the hospital. You obtain baseline vital signs and then contact medical control at the receiving facility to give your radio report. Once you have completed the report, you check to make certain that the patient is still resting comfortably. You then begin to write up the run report. The remainder of the call is uneventful.

1. How close should you hold the microphone to your lips for your voice to be picked up clearly and with minimal interference?
   - A. Pressed right against the microphone
   - B. 2" to 3"
   - C. 10" to 12"
   - D. At arm's length

2. Which of the following findings would **NOT** be considered an essential component of your radio report?
   - A. A complete family history of illnesses and injuries
   - B. The patient's chief complaint and response to treatment
   - C. The patient's level of responsiveness and vital signs
   - D. The treatment that has been provided for the patient

3. All of the following would be considered a part of the prehospital care communications system **EXCEPT**:
   - A. a portable radio.
   - B. a cellular telephone.
   - C. a repeater/base station.
   - D. a patient billing form.

4. You must ensure that your run report is written in:
   - A. black ink.
   - B. 15 minutes or less.
   - C. precise, organized fashion, according to local protocols.
   - D. complete detail, including everything that happened on the call.

5. A run report is **NOT** considered:
   - A. part of the patient's medical record.
   - B. a legal document.
   - C. a document that needs a signature.
   - D. necessary for nonemergency runs.

points to ponder

A lawsuit has been filed against you, your partner, and the ambulance service that you work for. It alleges negligence for your treatment of a 15-year-old patient. When your run report is pulled, it is incomplete, and your notes are very sketchy. You were providing patient care, and your partner filled out the report, but both of you signed it, as is normal protocol. In reviewing the case, you and your partner remember many of the issues differently from one another.

- How would you come to agreement on what was done? Would you complete the report now? What other records may be available to help clear up your differences? How could this have been prevented?

online outlook

The Federal Communications Commission (FCC) has five main EMS-related responsibilities. To learn more about the FCC's role in EMS, complete Exercise 9 at www.emtb.com.

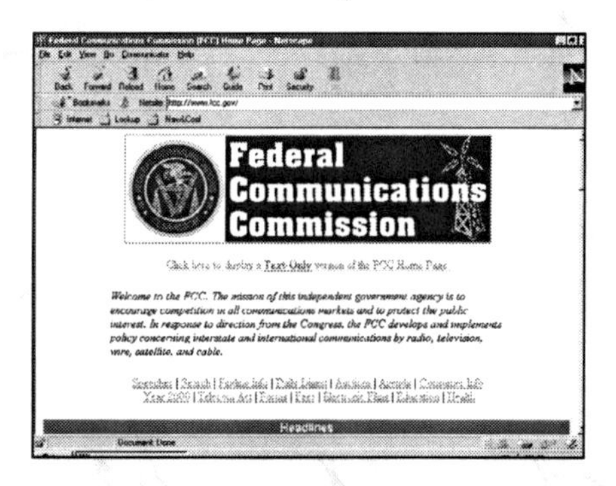

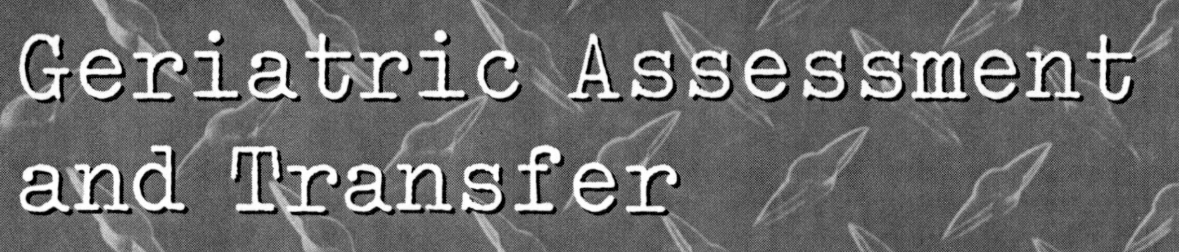

Geriatric Assessment and Transfer

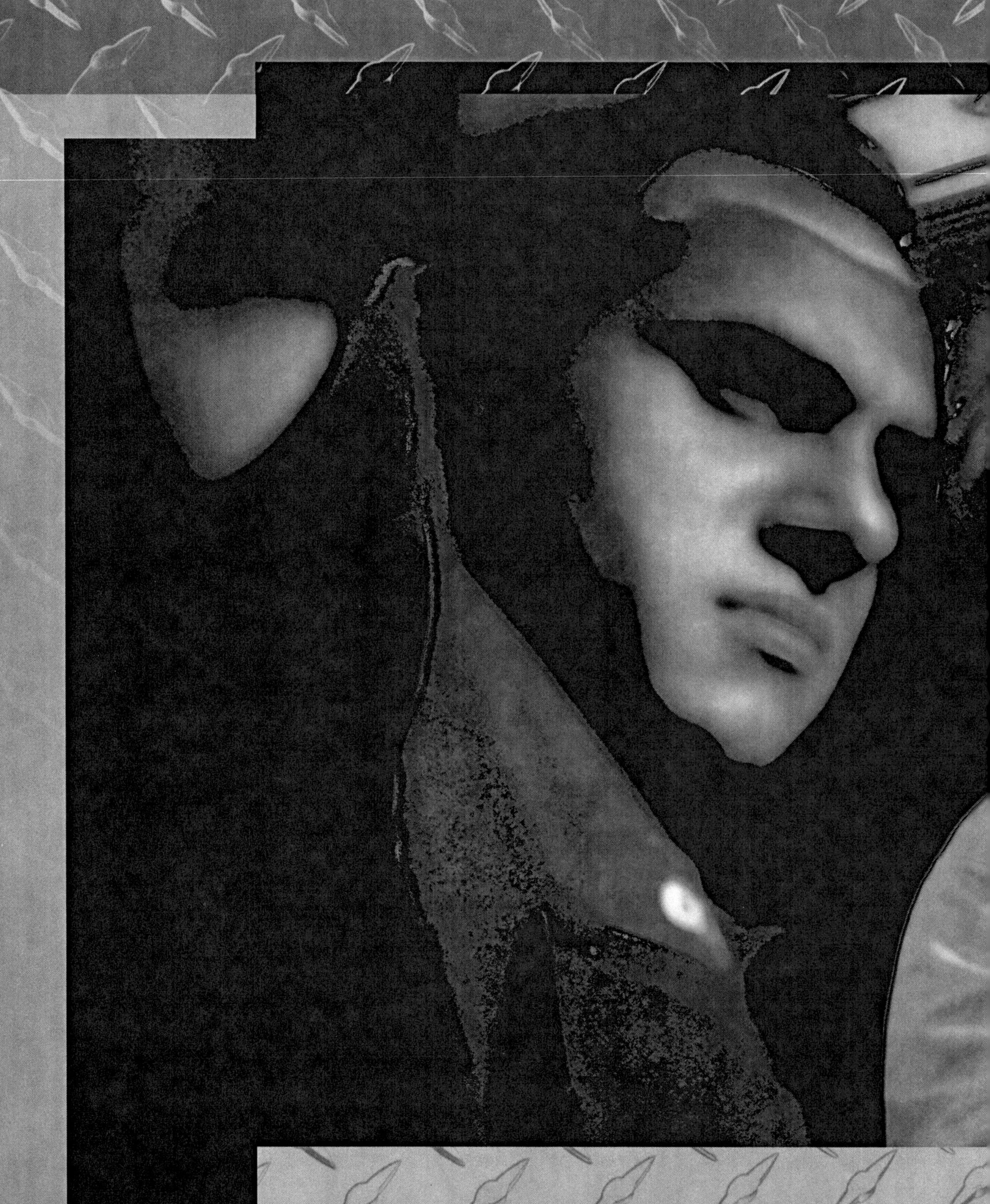

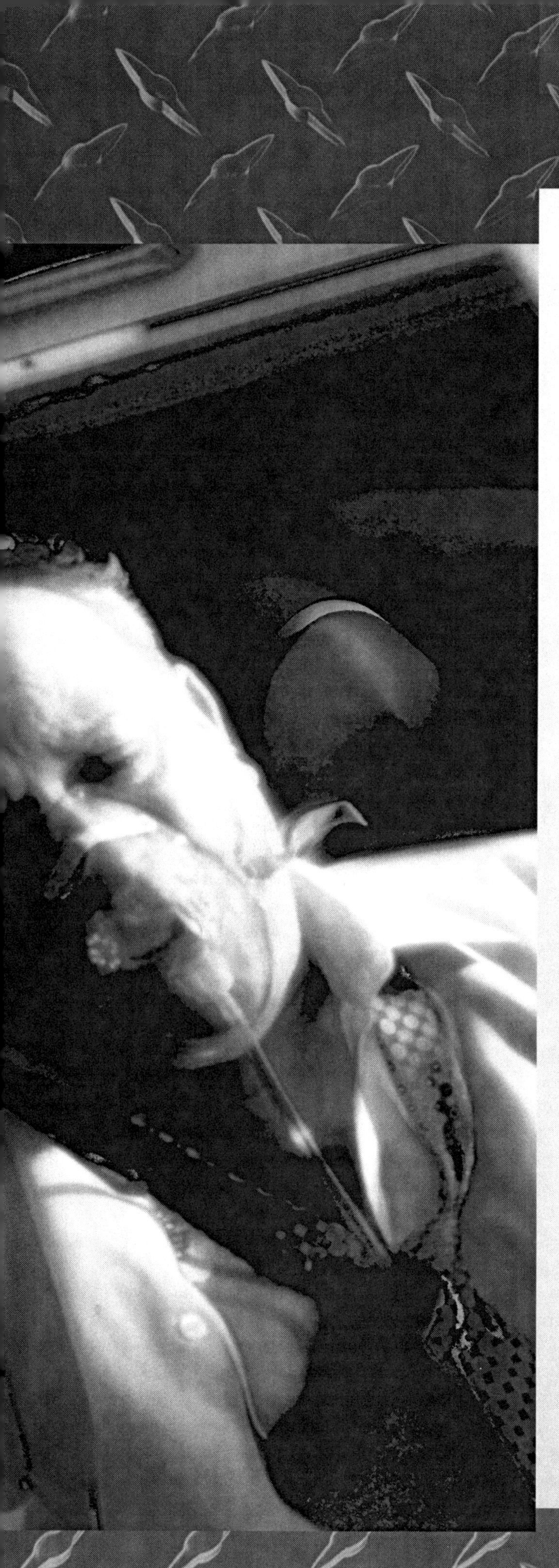

chapter 4

objectives*

Cognitive

1. Define the term "elderly."
2. State the leading causes of death of the elderly.
3. Describe the physiologic changes of aging.
4. Describe the following basics of patient assessment for the elderly:
   - Scene size-up
   - Initial assessment
   - Focused history and physical exam
5. Discuss response to elderly patients in nursing and skilled care facilities.
6. Describe trauma assessment in the elderly.
7. Describe acute illness assessment in the elderly for the following conditions:
   - Cardiovascular emergencies
   - Dyspnea
   - Syncope and altered mental status
   - Acute abdomen
8. State the principles and use of advance directives involving elderly patients.
9. Define elder abuse.
10. Discuss the causes of elder abuse.
11. Discuss why the extent of elder abuse is not well known.

Affective

12. Explain why the special needs of the elderly and the changes that the aging process brings about in physical structure, body composition, and organ function provide a fundamental knowledge base for maintenance of life support functions.

Psychomotor

13. Demonstrate the patient assessment skills that should be used to care for an elderly patient.

* These are non-curriculum objectives.

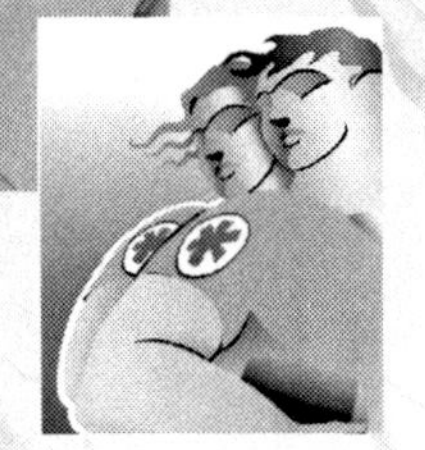

you are the cfr/emt

Rescue 6 please respond to Larson General Hospital to transfer a patient to Prairie View Nursing Home at 3200 Potter Road.

Although you may have taken the EMT course expecting to spend your days saving lives, many EMT-Bs who are new to the job will realize quickly that most EMS calls are for non-life-threatening emergencies or situations. Geriatric-related calls constitute a large portion of these calls, and the frequency of this type of call continues to increase. This chapter will prepare you to provide care for this challenging segment of society. It will also help you to answer the following questions:

1. Why do the signs, symptoms, and presentations of the ill or injured geriatric patient differ from those of other adults with similar problems?
2. What are some special transport considerations that might help to make the transfer of a geriatric patient an easier and less stressful experience?

Geriatric Assessment and Transfer

Geriatric or elderly patients are individuals who are older than age 65 years. No one relishes the thought of growing old, but the reality is that we all will, and the elderly will continue to make up a larger percentage of the population beyond the year 2000. According to the *1990 U.S. Census Data,* slightly more than 32 million individuals were older than age 65 years. By the year 2000, the elderly population will be roughly 35 million, and it is projected that by the year 2030, the elderly population will be greater than 70 million. This is a very significant evolutionary trend for the EMT-B because the elderly are major users of EMS and the health care system in general. The elderly use a disproportionate percentage of health care services and are more likely to call EMS. When they do call, their condition is likely to be serious, and they may not have the same type of "classic" presentation as younger patients. Their altered physiology may mask serious conditions. Elderly patients may also have a number of chronic medical problems and be taking numerous medications for their illnesses. Providing effective treatment for this growing number of patients will require that all EMT-Bs have an increased understanding of geriatric care issues and that they modify some of their assessment and treatment approaches.

While many EMT-Bs may relish the action of high-profile "knife-and-gun-club" calls, the reality is that the majority of your patient contacts will involve the elderly. Lifesaving interventions for geriatric patients may be as simple as noting the home environment, preventing falls, and making referrals to appropriate social services agencies. EMT-Bs who respond to the homes of elderly patients are in an ideal position not only to provide immediate help, but also to provide key information to others in the health care and social services systems. Often, simple preventive measures can help the elderly to avoid further injury, costly medical treatment, and death. The EMT-B is on the front line of helping to prevent and treat geriatric emergencies.

Leading Causes of Death

The leading cause of death in the elderly involves disease associated with the cardiovascular system, including heart disease and strokes. Trauma deaths among the elderly are usually associated with blunt trauma (motor vehicle crashes, motor vehicle versus pedestrians, falls) and penetrating trauma (gunshot wounds, knife wounds).

Table 10-1 shows the risk factors that affect mortality in elderly patients.

The elderly are more susceptible to disease and injury than are younger individuals. Acute illness or trauma is more likely to be accompanied by a chronic disease. In addition, acute illness and trauma are more likely to alter organ systems beyond those initially involved. For example, an elderly patient who has fallen and fractured a hip may also have a lung disorder.

TABLE 10-1 Risk Factors Affecting Mortality in Elderly Patients

- Age greater than 75 years
- Living alone
- Recent death of a significant other
- Recent hospitalization
- Incontinence (inability to hold urine or feces)
- Immobility
- Unsound mind

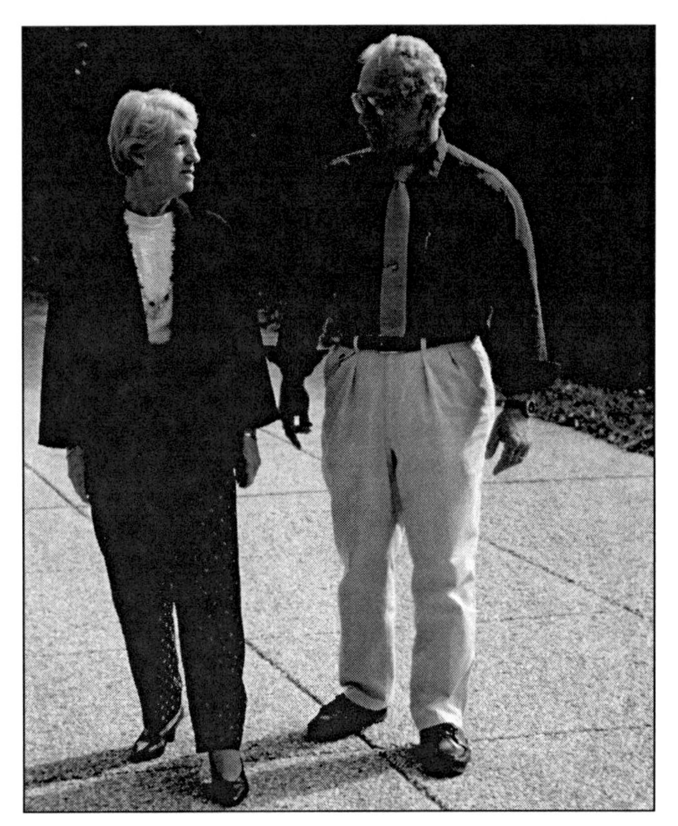

FIGURE 10-1 The elderly can continue to stay fit and active.

Physiologic Changes That Accompany Age

As we get older, our physiology changes. In general, a 65-year-old person cannot expect to have the same degree of physical performance as when he or she was 30 years old. By the time a person reaches age 65 years, the amount of total body water and the number of total body cells have decreased by as much as 30%. Generally, after age 30 years, organ systems begin to deteriorate at roughly 1% per year. However, the aging process does not necessarily mean disease.

As we age, even the very fit will experience the loss of ability to perform as well as they did when they were younger. The elderly can continue to stay fit and active even though they will not be able to perform at the same level as they did in their youth (Figure 10-1). Common stereotypes about the elderly include the presence of mental confusion, illness, a sedentary lifestyle, and immobility. Although these perceptions are common, they are usually very far from the norm. Most elderly individuals lead very active lives, participating in sports and in the community, and they are generally healthy in spite of the aging process. What happens when we age?

Skin

Collagen, which is the chief component of connective tissue and bones, is lost as we age, making the skin wrinkled, thinner, and more susceptible to injury. There are also fewer sweat glands, and the skin feels dry. Because it is less elastic, skin is more prone to laceration and bruising and generally takes longer to heal.

Senses

The pupils of the eyes begin to lose the ability to handle changes in light and require more time to adjust, which can make driving and walking more hazardous. Light changes can cause problems of visual acuity and depth perception. Cataracts, or clouding of the lenses, interfere with vision and make it difficult to distinguish colors and see clearly, increasing the likelihood of falls and accidents, as well as mistakes in taking various medications. Changes in the inner ear make hearing high-frequency sounds difficult; these changes can also cause problems with balance and make falls more likely. Changes in appetite may occur because of a decrease in the number of taste buds.

Respiratory System

Decreased elasticity in the lung tissue and a decreased lung surface area result in a decreased ability to exchange oxygen and carbon dioxide. In addition, the bronchial tree does not move mucous as well, increasing the chances of infection.

Cardiovascular System

Decreased cardiac output, an increased workload on the heart, and an accompanying decrease in the tolerance for exercise generally occur in the elderly. Many elderly patients are at risk for atherosclerosis, which is a disease of large- and medium-sized arteries in which fatty material is deposited and accumulates in the innermost

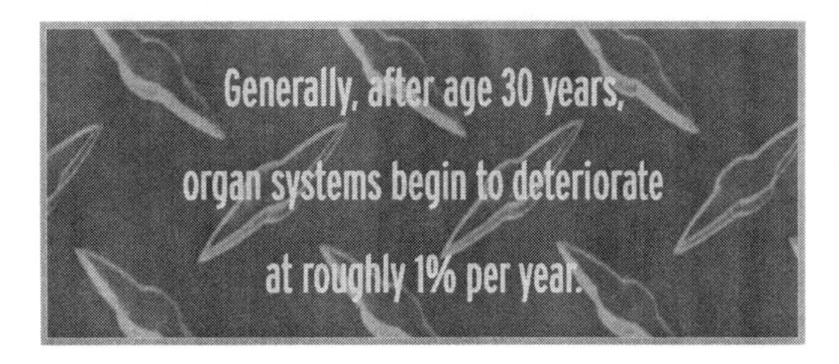

layer of the arteries. Major complications of atherosclerosis include myocardial infarction and stroke. The presence of arteriosclerosis, which is a disease that causes the arteries to thicken and harden, and calcification make stroke, heart disease, hypertension, and bowel infarction more likely. The elderly are also at an increased risk for aneurysm, an abnormal blood-filled dilation of the wall of a blood vessel, and catastrophic blood loss.

Renal System

Kidney function begins to decline because of a 30% to 40% decrease in functioning nephrons. With a decrease in renal function, electrolyte disturbances are more likely to occur. There is also a decrease in the amount of total body water.

Nervous System

The number of brain cells in some areas may decrease by as much as 45%. A 6% to 7% reduction in brain weight can result in memory impairment, a decrease in the ability to perform psychomotor skills, or slower reflex time. Brain shrinkage also makes the elderly individual more prone to head injury when a fall occurs.

Musculoskeletal System

The disks between the vertebrae begin to narrow, and a decrease in height of between 2" and 3" may occur. A decrease in the amount of muscle mass often results in less strength, and fractures are more likely to occur because of a decrease in bone density. Posture also changes as flexion at the knees, hips, and spine is more pronounced, making immobilization of the elderly more challenging.

Gastrointestinal System

A decrease in the volume of saliva and gastric juices causes a dry mouth, making it harder to chew and digest foods. Decreased liver function makes it harder to detoxify and eliminate substances such as drugs and alcohol.

Patient Assessment

Any time you assess a patient, you use the same basic approach: scene size-up, initial assessment, and a focused history and physical exam. Assessing an elderly patient is really no different. However, there are some issues that may indicate that you should modify your approach to the initial assessment or become more aware of some conditions that may affect the elderly patient.

The Basics

Your assessment of an elderly patient should include interviews with family members, friends, caretakers, senior citizen center workers, or significant others (Figure 10-2). You should remember that assessment of an elderly patient often takes longer and may be more difficult than that of a younger patient because of communication problems such as visual impairment, hearing loss, fatigue, and distractions in the immediate environment.

During assessment of an elderly patient, remember that the patient may have impaired hearing, sight, comprehension, and mobility. Try always to make eye contact, and grasp the patient's hand to feel for temperature, grip, and skin condition (Figure 10-3). Address the patient by his or her last name, using courtesy titles such as "Mr.," "Mrs.," or "Ms." Minimize noise, distractions, and interruptions.

During the assessment, you should observe the patient's behavior, dress and grooming, ease of rising and sitting, and fluency of speech. Watch for involuntary movement, cranial nerve dysfunction, and difficult respiration. Note whether the patient's movement is easy, unsteady, or unbalanced and whether the patient looks well nourished, thin, or emaciated.

Assessment of the elderly requires using different assessment skills than you would use for younger patients. Ask for specific rather than general information; the elderly tend to respond "yes" to all questions during the assessment process. Although asking open-ended questions is a useful tool when you are evaluating most patients, you may have to help an elderly patient by providing specific details to choose from. For example, "Describe the pain in your hip" and "Describe your chest pain " are open-ended and may lead to imprecise responses from the patient.

The following questions are more specific and may help the patient to give you better information:

- Is the pain in your hip sharp, stabbing, or dull?
- On a scale of 1 to 5, with 5 being the most intense pain, what number describes your pain?

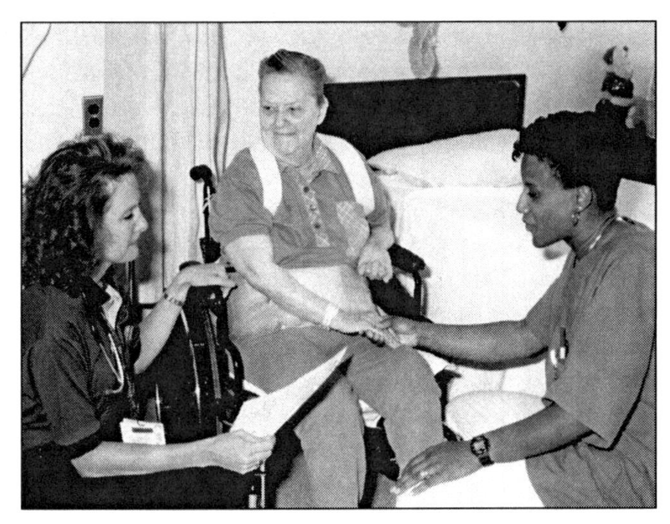

FIGURE 10-2 Interview family members, friends, and caretakers as part of your assessment of an elderly patient.

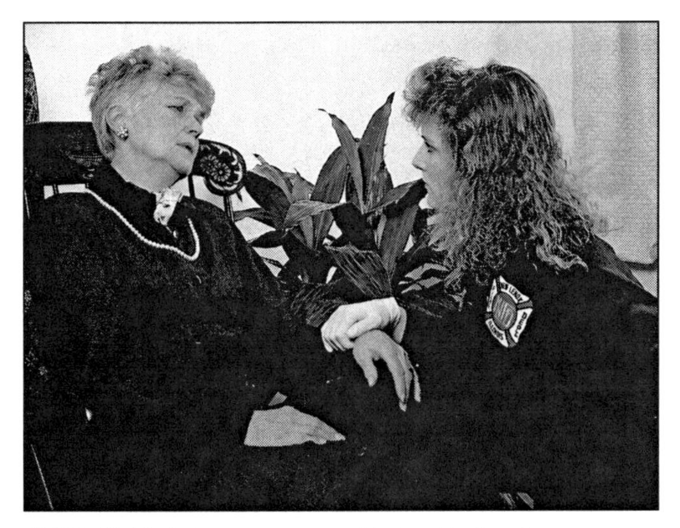

FIGURE 10-3 As you assess an elderly patient, make eye contact, and grasp the patient's hand to feel for temperature, grip, and skin condition.

Scene Size-Up

As you approach any scene, you must be keenly aware of the environment and the reason you were called. Activities of daily living such as the ability to move around, talk on the phone, prepare meals and eat, perform basic cleaning skills, and attend to personal hygiene are essential for continued health in all individuals. For the elderly, the aging or a disease process may make activities of daily living difficult and cause a spiral of problems. For example, suppose that a 70-year-old woman who trips on a loose floorboard is unable to regain her balance, falls, and dislocates her shoulder. She lives alone and has no one to help her with cooking and other daily activities. Her arm is treated, but in the following months of therapy, she becomes weaker and begins to have some difficulty walking, lifting even small objects, shopping, and making meals. She loses some weight and becomes weaker and is eventually forced to move to an adult care facility because of her need for constant help. All this was the result of a simple fall.

When you first arrive at a patient's residence, you should look for important clues to determine not only your safety, but also that of the occupant. The environment will provide a great deal of important information if you know what to look for.

The general condition of the home will give you some important clues. Is it being kept up, or are some serious repairs needed? Are there hazards, such as steep stairs, missing handrails, or other things that could cause a fall? Is it evident that the person may be having difficulty keeping the house clean? Is there some evidence of adequate food, water, heat, lights, and ventilation? Are there many pill bottles around, indicating treatment for some type of disease process? Does someone else live there who can help to answer questions? These are very important scene clues that can provide much information before you even contact the patient.

Initial Assessment

The sequence of the initial assessment is the same for pediatric, adult, and geriatric patients. However, you should not make any assumptions about an elderly patient's level of consciousness. Never assume that an altered mental status is normal. Altered mental status indicates some level of brain dysfunction and is a serious problem. The best rule of thumb is to always compare the patient's current level of consciousness or ability to function with the level or ability before the problem began. Do not assume that confusion or unresponsiveness is normal behavior for anyone. In many cases, you will have to rely on a family member or caretaker to help establish what the patient's baseline level of consciousness was before the complaint began.

During the initial assessment, you will assess the patient's complaint and ABC. If a life-threatening condition exists, you will have to perform emergency treatment before continuing your assessment. The initial assessment sets the tone and helps you to decide whether the patient requires a rapid resuscitative approach or a slower, contemplative one. In most cases, the slower, contemplative approach is all that is needed.

Focused History and Physical Exam

It is often said that 80% of a medical diagnosis is based on the patient's history. The history is usually the key in helping to assess a patient's problem. In addition to clearing the airway and managing the ABC, obtaining a coherent history is one of the most important things you can do. An inaccurate or inadequate history can cause you to make incorrect presumptions and pursue a flawed treatment plan.

To obtain an accurate history, patience and good communication skills are essential. An elderly patient's diminished sight, hearing, and speaking ability may hamper communications. If possible, take a few moments to get the patient's dentures, glasses, or hearing aid. All of these items can help the patient to communicate with you more effectively.

A poor history-gathering technique can hamper communications. You must be able to gain a patient's confidence, which is best accomplished by treating the patient with respect, taking a slow deliberate approach, and explaining what you are doing. First, ask the patient what his or her name is, and then use the patient's name. Avoid being overly familiar with the patient, and do not use any nicknames. Address the patient using courtesy titles, such as "Mr.," "Mrs.," or "Ms.," and his or her last name.

When there are multiple responders, there is a natural tendency to obtain a history "by committee." Everyone asks questions, sometimes several at a time. This is a poor technique that results in a haphazard history regardless of the patient's age. For elderly patients who may have communication or perceptual problems, it makes obtaining a coherent history almost impossible. In addition, many individuals are reluctant to discuss their problems in front of a crowd. Be sure to have one EMT-B obtain the patient's history, one question at a time, providing as much privacy as possible (Figure 10-4).

Reassure the patient, and use your best professional demeanor. Look at the patient when you are speaking, and be sure that the patient can see your lips. Use a normal tone of voice, especially if the patient is wearing a hearing aid. A loud tone may actually cause sound distortion in the hearing aid and make communication worse. Ask as many open-ended questions as possible, and use closed-ended questions to clarify points. While taking the history, write down any key points on a notepad so that you do not ask the same question repeatedly because you forgot the answer. Ask family members or caretakers to clarify what you just learned from the patient. Taking a few minutes to obtain an accurate history saves time in the long run by providing information on which accurate decisions can be based.

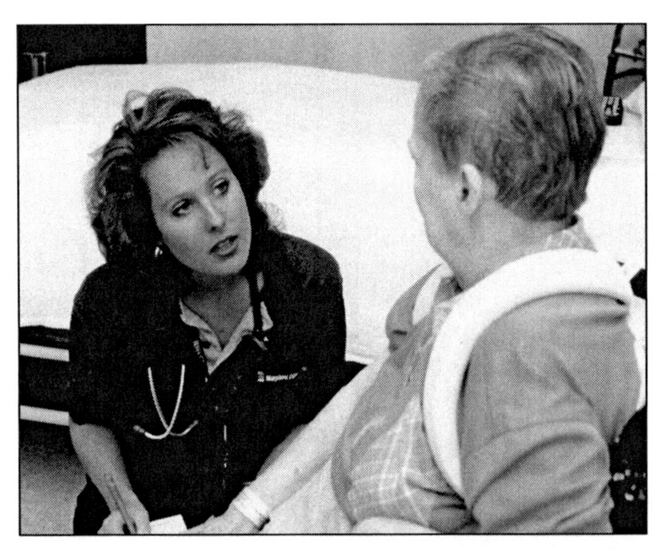

FIGURE 10-4 A slow, deliberate approach to the patient history, with one EMT-B asking the questions, is generally the best strategy in assessing an elderly patient.

Past medical conditions can provide information about the patient's current problem. If possible, enlist a family member or caretaker to write down the patient's past history. Elderly patients often suffer from more than one disease process at a time, and the symptoms of one disease may make the assessment of another more difficult.

Obtain a list of medications and dosages. Elderly patients are often prescribed multiple medications. Information about which medications are currently being taken is vital. In addition, find out whether the patient has recently started or stopped taking any of the medications. Medication interactions and noncompliance with instructions for taking prescribed drugs are common and may contribute to the patient's symptoms or problem.

Be aware that the sensation of pain may be diminished in an elderly patient, leading you to underestimate the severity of a condition. For example, 20% to 30% of elderly patients have "silent" heart attacks, without the typical symptom of chest pain. In addition, fear of hospitalization often causes the patient to either understate or minimize symptoms.

During the focused physical examination, be aware that elderly people are more prone to hypothermia than younger people are. Be sure to keep the patient warm and maintain the body temperature. Inspection and palpation can be hampered by multiple layers of clothing. Remove only the clothing that is necessary for examining the patient, and cover the patient back up when you are finished.

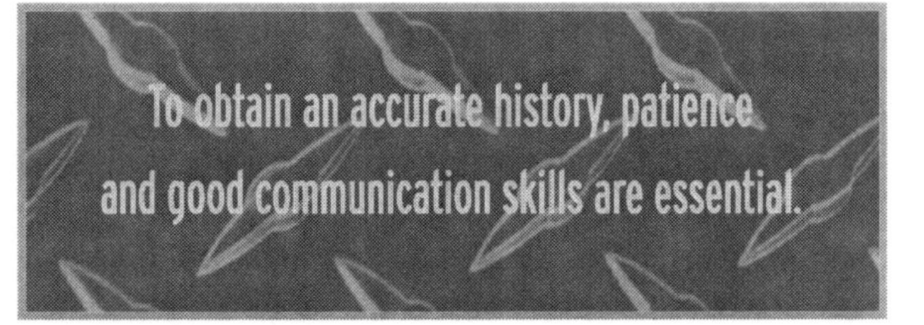

Response to Nursing and Skilled Care Facilities

Responding to a nursing home or skilled care facility is a common patient contact for EMT-Bs. Before you provide transport for the patient, you should find out the following critical information from the nursing staff:

- What is the patient's chief complaint today?
- What initial problem caused the patient to be admitted to the facility?

To determine the nature of the problem, you will usually have to compare the patient's present condition with his or her condition before onset of the symptoms. Ask the staff about the patient's mobility, activities of daily living, and ability to speak. This will help to paint a picture of the patient's baseline condition and indicate whether today's behavior differs from it.

Many facilities that are transferring patients will include a transfer record that contains the patient's history, medication lists and dosages, previous diagnosis, vital signs, allergies, and so on (Figure 10-5). These records provide members of the medical team with essential information and save time, especially when the patient cannot speak for himself or herself. Be sure to obtain this essential record before leaving for the hospital, and relay it to the hospital staff when giving your verbal report.

Trauma

Mechanism of Injury

Falls are the leading cause of trauma death and disability in the elderly. Most patients survive; however, a significant number require hospitalization. Motor vehicle trauma is the second leading cause of trauma death in the geriatric population. An elderly patient is five times more likely than a younger patient to be fatally injured in a car crash, even though excessive speed is rarely a causative factor in the older age group. Pedestrian accidents and burns are also common mechanisms of injury in elderly patients, resulting in death, serious injury, or disability.

Systemic Impact of Isolated Simple Trauma

You must also consider the body's decreasing ability to isolate simple trauma when you are assessing and caring for an elderly patient. An isolated hip fracture in a healthy 25-year-old adult is rarely associated with systemic decline. However, the same injury in an 85-year-old patient can produce a systemic impact that results in deterioration, shock, and life-threatening hypoxia, a dangerous condition in which the body tissues and cells do not have enough oxygen. Although an injury may be considered isolated and not alarming in most adults, an elderly patient's overall physical condition may have lowered the body's normal defenses

DEATON SPECIALTY HOSPITAL & HOME
611 South Charles Street
Baltimore, Maryland 21230
(410) 547-8500

PATIENT INFORMATION AND TRANSFER FORM

Name: ______ Date of Birth: ______ Sex: ___ Race: ______ Religion: ______
Social Security #: ______ Marital Status: M S W D Sep. Deaton Adm. Date: ______
Patient's Home Address: ______
Medicare #: ______ Medicaid #: ______ Other Ins.# ______
Responsible Party: ______ Relationship: ______ Home Phone: ______
Address: ______ Work Phone: ______

Date of Transfer: ______ Time: ______ Transferred To: ______
Unit Transferred From: ______ Nurse Manager: ______ Extension #: ______
Reason for Transfer: ______ Mode of Transport: ______
Physician in Charge at Time of Transfer: ______ Physician's Phone Number: ______

MAJOR DIAGNOSIS: ADVANCE DIRECTIVE: YES NO
CPR STATUS: ______

Vital Signs at Time of Transfer: BP: ______ Pulse: ______ Resp.: ______ Temp.: ______
Pertinent Medical Information: ______

Communicable Disease: YES NO Type: ______
Isolation: YES NO Type: ______
Suctioning: YES NO How Often: ______ Site: Oral ______ Trach ______
Ventilator Dependent: YES NO Vent Orders: ______

DRUGS AND OTHER THERAPY:
(at time of discharge)

Name	Frequency	Route

Diet Orders: ______
Method of Feeding: ______

LAB DATA
CXR: Date: ______ Result ______
CBC: Date: ______ Result ______

Form # 612 Rev. 9/94 Original Copy to go with Patient - Yellow Copy to be retained in Patient's Record

ADL'S	Independent	Needs Assistance	Unable to Do
Bed Activity: Turns / Sits			
Personal Hygiene:			
Feeding:			
Transfer: Sitting / Standing / Toilet			
Locomotion: Wheelchair / Walking			

Eyeglasses: YES NO Sent with pt.: YES NO
Dentures: YES NO Sent with pt.: YES NO

Patient Uses: ___ Cane ___ Crutches ___ Prosthesis ___ Walker ___ Chair ___ Stretcher
Bed Type: Side Rails: YES NO ___ Regular ___ Clinitron ___ Other ______
Usual Mental Status: (please circle) Alert Minimally Reactive Confused Forgetful Unresponsive
Communication Ability: Speech ___ Normal ___ Impaired Hearing ___ Normal ___ Impaired Appliance: YES NO
Incontinence: Bowel ___ Bladder ___ Colostomy ___ Catheter/Suprapubic ___

ADDITIONAL PERTINENT INFORMATION

ALLERGIES

Skin Condition:

Signature of Nurse Completing Transfer Form Date

NOTIFICATION TO EMERGENCY / TRANSPORTING PERSONNEL

This patient is diagnosed as having one of the following communicable diseases: (please circle)
1. HIV 2. Hepatitis B 3. Meningococcal Meningitis 4. Tuberculosis 5. Malaria 6. Rabies 7. Mononucleosis 8. NONE OF THE ABOVE
and is being transported to another facility - emergency or otherwise. Persons handling the transfer must be notified in writing by the transferring nurse of any of the above diseases. Disease notification must be made to:
- Law Enforcement Officer
- Firefighter
- Rescue Squad Personnel
- Emergency Medical Technician(s)

as required by the annotated Code of Maryland Article Health - General - Section 18-213-(D)-(2).

You are hereby notified . . . Signature of Nurse: ______ Date ______
Transport Representative: ______ Job Classification: ______ Date ______

Form # 612 Rev. 9/94 Original Copy to go with Patient - Yellow Copy to be retained in Patient's Record

FIGURE 10-5 A transfer record from a long-term care facility contains vital information for members of the medical team.

what do you think?

A cleaning service and a social worker sent by the city find an 80-year-old man, John, frozen to death in his second-floor apartment. For months, John's neighbors tried to help him because he did not seem to be able to care for himself. Neighbors gave him money for food and ran an extension cord to his apartment when his electricity was turned off. When John was found dead, the radiator in his apartment was working, but most of the heat was being lost through a broken window. The apartment was so cold that a half-empty can of beer near the window was frozen. Filthy clothing and sheets, soiled mattresses, and paint chips littered the apartment.

Jane is a 75-year-old woman with Alzheimer's disease who is confined to her apartment, where she lives with her husband, son, and daughter-in-law, Gail. Gail works full time as a waitress and provides most of Jane's support. Jane's 77-year-old husband, Bob, is retired and is a chronic alcohol abuser with a history of violence directed at his family. One morning, a neighbor sees a chair crash through the kitchen window and calls the police. The police find Gail unconscious on the kitchen floor and Jane bound and gagged on a mattress in the bedroom. Feces and urine are all over Jane's body. EMTs arriving at the scene find that the bed springs have broken Jane's skin. She also appears extremely malnourished and dehydrated.

Do you think John or Jane have been victims of elder abuse? Why or why not?

and ability to keep the effects of even a simple injury localized. Your assessment of the patient's condition and stability must include past medical conditions, even if they are not currently acute or symptomatic. For example, suppose you respond to a call about a patient with a history of unstable angina who sustains a simple isolated fracture of the ankle. You must consider this patient to be highly unstable and provide prompt transport before the stress and simple trauma worsen the angina and patient instability occurs.

Falls and Trauma

A medical condition such as fainting, a cardiac rhythm disturbance, or a medication interaction may lead to a fall that causes injury to the patient. Whenever you assess an elderly patient who has fallen, you must find out why the fall occurred. Did a fainting episode cause the fall and injury, or did the patient trip on something or lose his or her balance? Again, history is important. Sometimes, a recent history of starting or stopping blood pressure medication is enough to cause a patient to become dizzy and fall. Before you assume that the patient tripped before falling, obtain a careful history and bystander account. Consider that the fall may have been caused by a medical condition, and look carefully for clues from the patient, bystanders, and the environment. Although the trauma that the patient sustains from the fall can be serious, you should also consider that the medical condition that caused the fall may be life threatening.

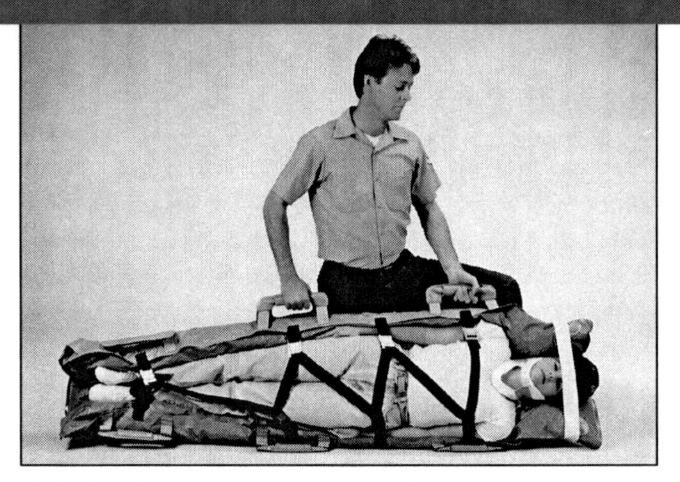

FIGURE 10-6 Vacuum mattresses that conform to body contours are a good choice for immobilizing the elderly.

When you respond to a motor vehicle crash, be alert to the possibility that a medical emergency may have caused the accident, especially in single vehicle collisions with no apparent cause.

Even if a patient has no life-threatening medical condition, injuries can lead to a downward spiral of loss of strength, mobility, and weakness, resulting in immobility and an inability to conduct activities of daily living.

Because brain tissue shrinks with age, the elderly are more likely to sustain closed head injuries, such as subdural hematomas. As a result of bone loss from osteoporosis, a generalized bone disease that is common among postmenopausal women, elderly patients are also prone to fractures, especially in areas such as the hip. With age, the spine stiffens as a result of shrinkage of disk spaces, and vertebrae become brittle. Fracture of the spine and spinal cord injuries are more likely to occur.

Because of the amount of flexion that occurs in the spinal column, hip, or knee of elderly patients, use of conventional splints and backboards to immobilize the patient may be difficult or impossible unless a lot of padding is used. What is considered a normal anatomic position for children and adults is often very abnormal for some elderly trauma patients. You should try to determine the patient's baseline condition and what was normal for the patient before the accident. Trying to force a patient with pronounced joint flexion into "normal" anatomic position can be very painful for the patient and frustrating for you. Some devices, such as traction splints, simply do not work on patients with flexed hips and knees. Splinting devices, such as vacuum mattresses that conform to body contours, may be a better choice for immobilization than a conventional backboard (Figure 10-6).

Remember that when you treat an elderly trauma patient, you must assess the injuries and carefully look for the cause of the fall or crash.

Cardiovascular Emergencies

Syncope

You should always assume that syncope, or fainting, in the elderly is a life-threatening problem until proven otherwise. Syncope is caused by an interruption of blood flow to the brain. Syncope has many causes; some are serious and others are not. Either way, an elderly person who has a period of unconsciousness should be examined to determine the cause of the syncope. Table 10-2 shows some of the causes of syncope in an elderly patient.

Heart Attack

The classic symptoms of a heart attack are often not present in the elderly. As many as one-third of elderly patients have "silent" heart attacks in which the usual chest pain is not present. Table 10-3 shows signs and symptoms that are commonly noted in elderly patients who are experiencing a heart attack.

TABLE 10-2 Possible Causes of Syncope in an Elderly Patient

Cardiac Dysrhythmias/ Dysrhythmias/ Heart Attack	The heart is beating too fast or too slowly, the cardiac output drops, and blood flow to the brain is interrupted. A heart attack can also cause syncope.
Vascular and Volume	Medication interactions can cause venous pooling and vasodilation, a widening of the blood vessel, resulting in a drop in blood pressure and inadequate blood flow to the brain. Another cause can be a drop in blood volume because of hidden bleeding from a condition such as an aneurysm.
Neurologic	A transient ischemic attack or a "brain attack" can sometimes mimic syncope.

TABLE 10-3 Common Signs and Symptoms of Heart Attack in an Elderly Patient

Dyspnea	Dyspnea, the feeling of shortness of breath or difficulty in breathing, is a common complaint in the elderly and is most often associated with heart attack. It is often combined with other symptoms, such as nausea, weakness, and sweating. Chest pain associated with angina typically has an onset during periods of stress or exertion. In the elderly, chest pain is often not present, but exertional dyspnea is. As the disease progresses, dyspnea may have an onset without exertion. Dyspnea in the elderly is often the equivalent of chest pain in younger patients who are having angina or a heart attack. In addition, congestive heart failure and acute pulmonary edema may result from the "silent" heart attack.
A Weak Feeling	Weakness can be caused by many things. However, you should suspect a heart attack in a patient with a sudden onset of weakness. Weakness is often associated with sweating.
Syncope/Confusion/ Altered Mental Status	Syncope can have many causes, and in the elderly, none of these causes should be presumed to be minor. Major life-threatening causes of syncope are often cardiac in origin. Altered mental status is usually a signal of poor blood supply to the brain, often from cardiac dysrhythmia and heart attack.

The Acute Abdomen

A number of life-threatening abdominal catastrophes are common in elderly patients. Because of pain referral patterns and the possibility that the patient does not feel any pain, abdominal complaints in the elderly are notoriously difficult to assess. In the field, the one result of abdominal catastrophe is blood loss, which leads to shock and death. *Abdominal aortic aneurysm* (AAA) is one of the most rapidly fatal conditions. AAA tends to develop in individuals who have a history of hypertension and atherosclerosis.

Elderly patients are also more prone to abdominal problems because of the loss of collagen, which makes vessels and connective tissue weaker. The walls of the aorta weaken, and blood begins to leak into the layers of the vessel, causing the aorta to bulge like a bubble on a tire. If enough blood is lost into the vessel wall itself, shock occurs. If the wall bursts, it rapidly leads to fatal blood loss. When the problem is caught early, there is a chance to repair the vessel before rupture and fatal blood loss occur.

A patient with an abdominal aortic aneurysm most commonly reports abdominal pain radiating through to the back with occasional flank pain. If the AAA becomes large enough, it can be felt as a pulsating mass in the midline of the abdomen during physical examination. Occasionally, the AAA causes a decrease in blood flow to one of the iliac arteries, and the patient complains of some discomfort in the affected extremity. Assessment may also reveal diminished or absent pulses in the extremity. Compensated shock (early shock) and decompensated shock (late shock) as a result of blood loss are common occurrences. Because of a decrease in blood volume and decreased blood flow to the brain, the patient may experience syncope. You should treat the patient for shock and provide prompt transport to the hospital.

Another cause of abdominal pain and shock is gastrointestinal bleeding, which can occur for a variety of reasons and is usually heralded by the vomiting of blood or material that looks like coffee grounds. Bleeding in the lower digestive tract is usually manifested by black or tarry stools. A patient with gastrointestinal bleeding may experience weakness, dizziness, or syncope. Bleeding into the gastrointestinal system can be life threatening because of the potential for blood loss and shock.

Altered Mental Status

Because of our stereotypical perceptions about the elderly, we may expect them to forget names or not be able to remember events or learn new things. However, these types of changes in mental status are not part of the normal aging process. They may be part of a slow deterioration or a condition or disease of rapid onset, neither of which is normal. To determine the onset of this change in mental status, you must compare the patient's ability to function with that of the recent past. This will help to establish a baseline and give some perspective on the onset of the change. The two terms that are often used to describe a change in mental status are "delirium" and "dementia."

Delirium is a change in mental status that is marked by the inability to focus, think logically, and maintain attention. Acute anxiety may be present in addition to the other symptoms. Usually, memory remains mostly intact. Delirium is commonly marked by an acute or recent onset and is a "red flag" for some type of new health problem. Delirium may be caused by tumors, fever, or drug or alcohol intoxication or withdrawal. Delirium can be present from metabolic causes as well. Any time a patient has an acute onset of delirious behavior, you should rapidly assess the patient for the following three conditions:

- Hypoxia
- Hypovolemia
- Hypoglycemia

Any of these three conditions, if left unrecognized or untreated, may be rapidly fatal.

Dementia is the slow onset of progressive disorientation, shortened attention span, and loss of cognitive function. Dementia develops slowly over a period of years rather than a few days. Alzheimer's disease, brain attacks, or genetic factors may cause dementia. Dementia is usually considered irreversible and is an expected course of the pathophysiologic neurologic disease process. The patient's history and determination of function in the recent past are key factors in determining the baseline. Delirium is caused by emergent problems; dementia is not.

Advance Directives

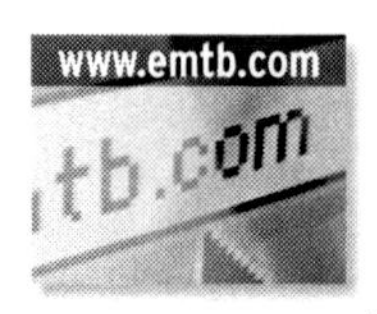

Many individuals today are making use of advance directives, specific legal papers that direct relatives and caregivers about what kind of medical treatment may be given to them if they cannot speak for themselves. An advance directive is also commonly called a living will. It can also take the form of "Do not resuscitate" (DNR) orders and health care proxies. DNR orders give you permission *not* to attempt resuscitation. However, for a DNR order to be valid, the patient's medical problems must be clearly stated, and the form must be signed by the patient or legal guardian and by one or more physicians. The form must be dated within the preceding 12 months. Even in the presence of a DNR order, you are still obligated to provide supportive measures, such as oxygen, pain relief, and comfort when you can.

A health care proxy is exercised by an individual who has been authorized by the patient to make medical decisions for the patient. Be sure to follow your service's protocol when faced with an advance directive.

Mentally competent adults and emancipated minors have the right to consent to or decline treatment, provided that they are competent to do so. The definition of competence is often hotly debated, but a person who is older than 18 years of age, alert, and not intoxicated and who understands the consequences of his or her decision is generally deemed competent. Unfortunately, patients who are unconscious or in a medical crisis are not able to inform medical personnel about their wishes to consent to or decline treatment. It is dangerous to take someone else's word for what the patient's wishes are; this is the reason that written advance directives have been developed.

Dealing with advance directives has become more common for EMS providers as more individuals are electing to use hospice services and spend their final days at home. Although advance directives may be in place, family members or caregivers who are present at the time of death or when the patient's condition worsens often become alarmed and call 9-1-1. Family members and caretakers may then become upset when you take resuscitative action and begin transportation to the hospital.

Another common situation is the transportation of patients from nursing facilities. Specific guidelines vary from state to state; however, you should consider the following general guidelines:

- Patients have the right to refuse treatment, including resuscitative efforts, provided that they are able to communicate their wishes.
- A DNR order is valid in a health care facility only if it is in the form of a written order by a physician.
- You should periodically review state and local protocols and legislation regarding advance directives.
- When you are in doubt or when there are no written orders, you should try to resuscitate the patient.

It is absolutely essential that every EMT-B becomes familiar with his or her state regulations regarding advance directives. Every service should also provide additional training on the actions you should take when presented with advance directives. When in doubt, your best course of action is to take resuscitative action that is appropriate to the situation and to practice sound medical treatment.

Elder Abuse

Reports and complaints of abuse, neglect, and other related problems among the nation's elderly are on the rise. The exact extent of elder abuse is not known for several reasons, including the following:

- Elder abuse is a problem that has been largely hidden from society.
- The definitions of abuse and neglect among the elderly vary.
- Victims of elder abuse are often hesitant to report the problem to law enforcement agencies or human and social welfare personnel.

In 1981, The House Select Committee on Aging concluded that 4% of the elderly nationwide, or more than 1.1 million individuals, were victims of some kind of abuse.

A parent who feels ashamed or guilty because he or she raised the abuser is often a typical victim of elder abuse. The abused individual may also feel traumatized by the situation or be afraid that the abuser will try to get back at him or her. In some areas of the country, there is a lack of formal reporting mechanisms, and some states lack statutory provisions that require that elder abuse be reported.

The physical and emotional signs of abuse, such as rape, spouse beating, or nutritional deprivation, are often overlooked or not accurately identified. Older women in particular are not likely to report incidents of sexual assault to law enforcement agencies. Patients with sensory deficits, senility, and other forms of altered mental status, such as drug-induced depression, may not be able to report abuse.

Elder abuse is defined as any action on the part of an elderly individual's family member, caretaker, or other associated person that takes advantage of the elderly individual's person, property, or emotional state; it is also called *granny battering* or *parent battering*.

The elderly individual who is likely to be abused is generally older than 65 years of age. Elder abuse occurs most often in women older than 75 years of age. The abused person is often frail with multiple chronic medical conditions, has dementia, and may suffer from an impaired sleep cycle, sleepwalking, and periods of shouting at others. The individual may be incontinent and in general is dependent on others for activities of daily living.

Abusers of the elderly are often products of child abuse themselves, and the abuse that is inflicted upon the elderly may be a retaliatory matter. As with cases of child and spousal abuse, if the family history indicates patterns of abuse or weak family ties, or if children have been ill treated or treated violently, the probability of elder abuse is greater. Because many elderly individuals live in a family environment and are typically women older than 75 years of age, you must try to find clues from the environment. The abuser is frequently the spouse or a middle-aged daughter-in-law who is caring for dependent children and dependent parents while perhaps holding full- or part-time employment. Most of these abusers are not trained in the particular care that the elderly require and have little relief time from the constant care demands of their own family, children, and spouse. Their lives are now complicated by the often less-than-flexible elderly individual they have to care for.

The abuser may also suffer from marked fatigue, be unemployed with financial difficulties, and be a substance abuser.

Abuse is not restricted to the home; environments such as nursing, convalescent, and continuing care centers are also sites where the elderly sustain physical, chemical, or pharmacologic harm. Often, care providers in these environments consider the elderly to represent management problems or categorize them as obstinate and undesirable patients. When called to the scene to treat an elderly patient who you suspect may have been abused, you may find that elder abuse can be gruesome, vulgar, barbaric, or worse than that inflicted upon children.

Assessment of Elder Abuse

While assessing the patient, you should try to obtain an explanation of what happened. You should suspect abuse when frank answers to questions about what caused the injury are concealed or avoided.

You must also suspect abuse when you are given unbelievable answers from anyone other than the patient, the possible abuser, or significant witnesses. Answers to questions you ask such as "Exactly where did this happen?," "Exactly what was the patient doing?," and "What time did it happen?" may provide valuable clues to whether the patient was abused. You should be suspicious if you think "Does this make sense?" or "Do I really believe this story?" while reviewing the patient's history. If you see burns, especially cigarette burns or physical marks that indicate that certain parts of the patient's body have been scalded systematically, you must also suspect abuse. As an EMT-B, you may be the first health care provider to observe possible abuse. You should try to find out information related to violent incidents when gathering the patient's medical history. Information that may be important in assessing possible abuse includes the following:

- Repeated visits to the emergency department or clinic
- A history of being "accident prone"
- Soft-tissue injuries
- Unbelievable or vague explanations of injuries
- Psychosomatic complaints
- Chronic pain
- Self-destructive behavior
- Eating and sleep disorders
- Depression or a lack of energy
- Substance and/or sexual abuse

You should remember that many patients suffering abuse are so afraid of retribution that they make false statements. An elderly patient who is being abused by family members may lie about the origin of abuse for fear of being removed from the home. In other cases of elder abuse, sensory deprivation or dementia may hinder adequate explanation.

Your assessment of the patient is important, not only to identify abuse that may not be reported by the patient, but also to uncover pathology. A physician may have to diagnose some abuse cases with X-rays or magnetic resonance imagery. You can observe other abuse, such as malnutrition, by visual examination; you can discover such abuse as swelling of an extremity by palpation.

In addition to the lifesaving care that you can provide the patient, your examination of the patient can help to reduce further trauma from abuse through its very identification. Repeated abuse can lead to a high risk of death. A preventive measure in reducing additional maltreatment of the patient is identification of the abuse by emergency medical providers. This may allow for referral and protective services of human, social, and public safety agencies (Table 10-4).

TABLE 10-4 Categories of Elder Abuse

Category	Examples
Physical	• Assault • Neglect • Dietary • Poor maintenance of home • Poor personal care
Psychological	• Benign neglect • Verbal • Being treated as an infant • Deprivation of sensory stimulation
Financial	• Theft of valuables • Embezzlement

Signs of Physical Abuse

Signs of abuse may be quite obvious or subtle. Obvious signs include bruises; burns; head, chest, abdominal, or bone injuries; and sexual abuse injuries. Subtle signs include undernourishment or a failure to thrive. You must record and document your findings when you examine the patient.

Inflicted bruises are usually found on the buttocks and lower back, genitals and inner thighs, cheeks or earlobes, upper lip and inside the mouth, and neck. Pressure bruises caused by the human hand may be identified by oval grab marks, pinch marks, hand prints, linear marks, or bruises that encircle the trunk. Human bites are typically inflicted on the upper extremities. Human bites can cause lacerations, crushing, and infection.

You should also investigate multiple bruises in various states of healing by questioning the patient and reviewing the patient's activities of daily living.

Burns are a common form of abuse. Most of these burns are not examined in a medical setting. Typical abuse from burns are caused by contact with cigarettes, matches, heating devices, heated metal, forced immersion in hot liquids, chemicals, and electrical power sources.

Your assessment of a patient who has been burned should include attention to burns that may cause airway distress, especially facial burns, burned sputum, and singeing of facial and nasal hair.

As in all abuse cases, you should obtain a history of the injury, especially in burn cases. Pay special attention to the need for life support measures. Burns can lead to death in many elderly patients. Be sure to observe the patient's body for blisters, fresh burns, and imprints of items such as a hot poker or iron. Remove any jewelry from the patient's arm or hand to prevent constriction.

Injuries to the head from direct blows are generally a high cause of mortality in abused patients. Pay special attention to the ABC in patients who have received a head injury.

Specific head injuries include blows, lacerations, and pulling of hair from the scalp. Because of the scalp's abundant blood supply, significant blood loss can occur. Blunt trauma, impalement injuries, and bullet wounds to the head can lead to subdural hematomas. Bleeding from the nose, wounds or burns of the lips and tongue, missing or loose teeth, broken bones in the face, and bruises in the corners of the mouth may indicate abuse.

Damage to the eyes is of particular concern in cases of elder abuse. Was there blunt or penetrating trauma? Were chemicals involved?

You should also inspect the patient's ears for indications of twisting, pulling, or pinching or evidence of frequent blows to the outer ears.

The chest is often an area of assault. Be sure to inspect the patient's chest for evidence of blunt or penetrating trauma. Blunt trauma may result from a hit with a baseball bat, a fist, or a hard bar of soap wrapped in a towel. Penetrating trauma may be evident from sharp instruments such as an ice pick, knife, or screwdriver. Elderly individuals may be restrained by the abuser with various tie devices that can result in rib fractures or internal damage to organs in the thoracic cage. You must immediately treat any impairment of breathing.

Injury to organs in the abdominal cavity are serious and may be life threatening. Blunt and penetrating trauma are the usual mechanisms of injury; however, poisoning or forced ingestion of caustic substances may be involved. Damage to the internal organs may be caused by blows from the back of a fist. Unrecognized abdominal injury can lead to death.

Be sure to examine the extremities for bruises or deformity, in addition to distal circulation. Ordinarily, fractures are not life threatening; however, multiple fractures to the femur or pelvis can lead to blood loss and death.

It may be difficult to see a failure to thrive in an elderly patient who has been abused. You should observe the patient's weight and try to determine whether the patient appears undernourished or has been unable to gain weight in the current environment. Does the patient have a ravenous appetite? Has medication been withheld? Is money being withheld, so the patient cannot buy food or medicine? You should also check for signs of neglect, such as evidence of a lack of hygiene, poor dental hygiene, poor temperature regulation or lack of reasonable amenities in the home.

You must regard injuries to the genitals or rectum with no reported trauma as evidence of sexual abuse in any patient. Elderly patients with altered mental status may never be able to report sexual abuse. In addition, many women do not report cases of sexual abuse because of shame and the pressure to forget. Sexually abused patients often have difficulty reporting the violence, so you must carefully scrutinize and review implausible explanations.

Renal injury may occur from blunt trauma to the flank or back, indicated by contusions, hematomas, or ecchymosis. Perforation of the ureter and bladder may result from penetrating trauma.

Lacerations, bruises, or injury to the genitalia, incontinence, and evidence of sexually transmitted disease or other infection must raise the question in your mind as to the cause.

prep kit

ready for review

Management of elderly patients can present you with many challenges that are not encountered with younger patients and confront you with a host of different problems that may be quite difficult and frustrating to solve. The health problems of the elderly are multifaceted, and frequent barriers to communication can be expected. In managing the elderly patient, things may not be packaged in their normal framework.

Although assessment of the elderly patient involves the same basic approach as with any other patient, you must take a more wary approach to the elderly patient. The injury or medical condition may be worse than is indicated by the existing signs and symptoms, and the injuries and conditions that are found will have a more profound effect than they would in a younger patient. You should also note that in addition to the critical needs that an underlying medical problem may cause, the elderly patient may be more unstable than a younger patient, thus having an increased possibility for sudden rapid deterioration.

The exact extent of elder abuse is not known because many patients do not report it. Victims of elder abuse are generally women older than 65 years of age. Abusers are often family members who must care for the elderly person in addition to caring for their own spouses and children. Elder abuse also occurs in nursing, convalescent, and continuing care centers. Elder abuse can be gruesome, vulgar, and barbaric, and is often worse than abuse inflicted on children. You must provide lifesaving care to the patient and also try to reduce additional abuse through identification of the problem. Identification of abuse by emergency medical providers can lead to referral and protective services of human, social, and public safety agencies.

Remember, the elderly patient you are caring for has made it to this age. Whether because of better medical care, genetics, or some other factor, the patient has survived. Growing old is not easy work, and neither is the emergency medical care of the elderly patient. You must be careful to obtain an accurate history of the patient, be patient, and communicate effectively. The duty that we owe to our elders and the sense of service provided to them is one of our more important callings.

vital vocabulary

www.emtb.com

advance directives Written documentation that specifies medical treatment for a competent patient should he or she become unable to make decisions.

aneurysm An abnormal blood-filled dilation of a blood vessel.

atherosclerosis A disease in which fatty material is deposited and accumulates in the innermost layer of medium- and large-sized arteries.

arteriosclerosis A disease that is characterized by hardening and thickening of the arterial walls.

cataract Clouding of the lens of the eye or its surrounding transparent membrane.

collagen A protein that is the chief component of connective tissue fibrils and bones.

compensated shock Early shock.

decompensated shock Late shock.

delirium A change in mental status marked by the inability to focus, think logically, and maintain attention.

dementia The slow onset of progressive disorientation, shortened attention span, and loss of cognitive function.

dyspnea Shortness of breath or difficulty breathing.

elder abuse Any action on the part of an elderly individual's family member, caretaker, or other associated person that takes advantage of the elderly individual's person, property, or emotional state; also called *granny battering* or *parent battering*.

hypoxia A dangerous condition in which the body tissues and cells do not have enough oxygen.

osteoporosis A generalized bone disease that is common among postmenopausal women in which there is a reduction in the amount of bone mass, leading to fractures after minimal trauma.

syncope Fainting caused by an interruption of blood flow to the brain.

vasodilation Widening of a blood vessel.

assessment **in action**

You and your partner are called to a private residence for a woman who had fallen. Upon arrival, you are met at the door by the patient, an 83-year-old woman. She states that she does not think she needs an ambulance but her neighbor, who was visiting at the time she fell, insisted on calling 9-1-1. You find out that the woman actually fell about an hour ago. She landed squarely on her buttocks.

You note that the patient is limping markedly, but your assessment reveals only minimal swelling and no obvious deformity. The patient is alert and oriented but appears very pale. She has a blood pressure of 88/70 mm Hg, a pulse of 58 beats/min, and respirations of 26 breaths/min.

As you and your partner lift the patient onto the stretcher, she cries out in pain, and you now note an obvious, significant deformity just below her right hip. Test results at the hospital reveal that she has a blood alcohol level of 0.282 and a fractured right hip.

1. Which of the patient's vital signs is within normal limits for her age group?
   A. Pulse
   B. Skin color
   C. Respirations
   D. Blood pressure
2. Assessment of a patient with a suspected fracture of the hip should **NOT** include an evaluation of the patient's:
   A. ability to bear weight or walk.
   B. ability to move the toes on the injured extremity.
   C. ability to feel sensations distal to the injury.
   D. skin color and distal pulses in the injured extremity.
3. Which of the following statements about fractures of the hip is true?
   A. Distal circulation is usually not affected.
   B. Swelling and deformity of the extremity are often absent.
   C. The patient may be able to stand and walk.
   D. Internal rotation of the affected foot is a common presentation.
4. Which of the following statements about alcohol intoxication in the elderly is true?
   A. Alcohol intoxication may alter pain sensation.
   B. An alcohol odor on the breath may be present but overlooked.
   C. Elderly patients from lower income socioeconomic groups are more likely to be alcoholics.
   D. Increased liver function in the elderly easily eliminates alcohol from the patient's system.
5. What is the most likely reason the EMT-Bs overlooked the possibility that the patient was intoxicated?
   A. The patient would have had flushed skin if she were intoxicated.
   B. The patient would have had a higher blood pressure if she were intoxicated.
   C. The patient would have shown obvious signs of alcohol use.
   D. The patient would have been vomiting if she were intoxicated.

points **to ponder**

You respond to a call about an elderly man with severe abdominal pain. When you arrive, his wife lets you in and tells you that she called for you. She says that he has had pain for about three hours now. You find the man sitting at the kitchen table. He is wearing very thick glasses and asks who is there as you walk into the room. It is obvious that his vision is very poor. As you begin talking to him, you find out that he is also quite deaf. You must yell to him to communicate, and at that, he appears to hear only about one-third of what you are saying. He appears confused and disoriented, but you are not sure whether that is mental or because he cannot see or hear very well. He is complaining about pain in his feet. He says that he does have abdominal pain, but mostly it is his feet. His feet feel cold and are a little cyanotic, but both are about the same. His wife insists that he was having severe abdominal pain earlier. When you ask about medications, he produces a shoe box with about 20 pill bottles, 12 of which he says he takes at least once a week. You find yourself very frustrated with the lack of information you are able to obtain.

- How would you treat this man? Would you transport him? How else could you get more information? He is not refusing care, but it is unclear whether he needs it. On what would you base your decisions?

online **outlook**

In order to provide effective treatment to the growing number of elderly patients, all EMTs must have an increased understanding of geriatric care issues. Learn more about the health of geriatric Americans by completing Exercise 10 at www.emtb.com.

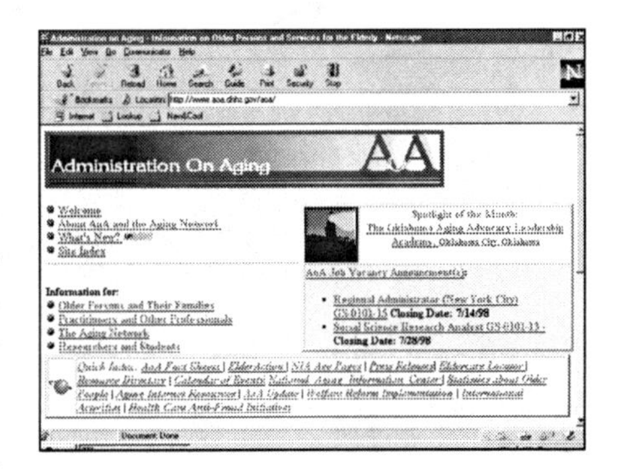

Photo Credits

Chapter 1

8-4: Reproduced with permission of the Maryland Institute of Emergency Medical Services Systems (MIEMSS), 8-8: © J. Higgins, Unicorn Stock Photos, 8-9: © Linda Gheen

Chapter 3

9-14: © Lawrence Migdale, Photo Researchers, inc., 9-15: © Linda Gheen

Chapter 4

Opener: © Bruce Ayers, Tony Stone Images
10-6: Courtesy of Hartwell Medical

Notes

Notes

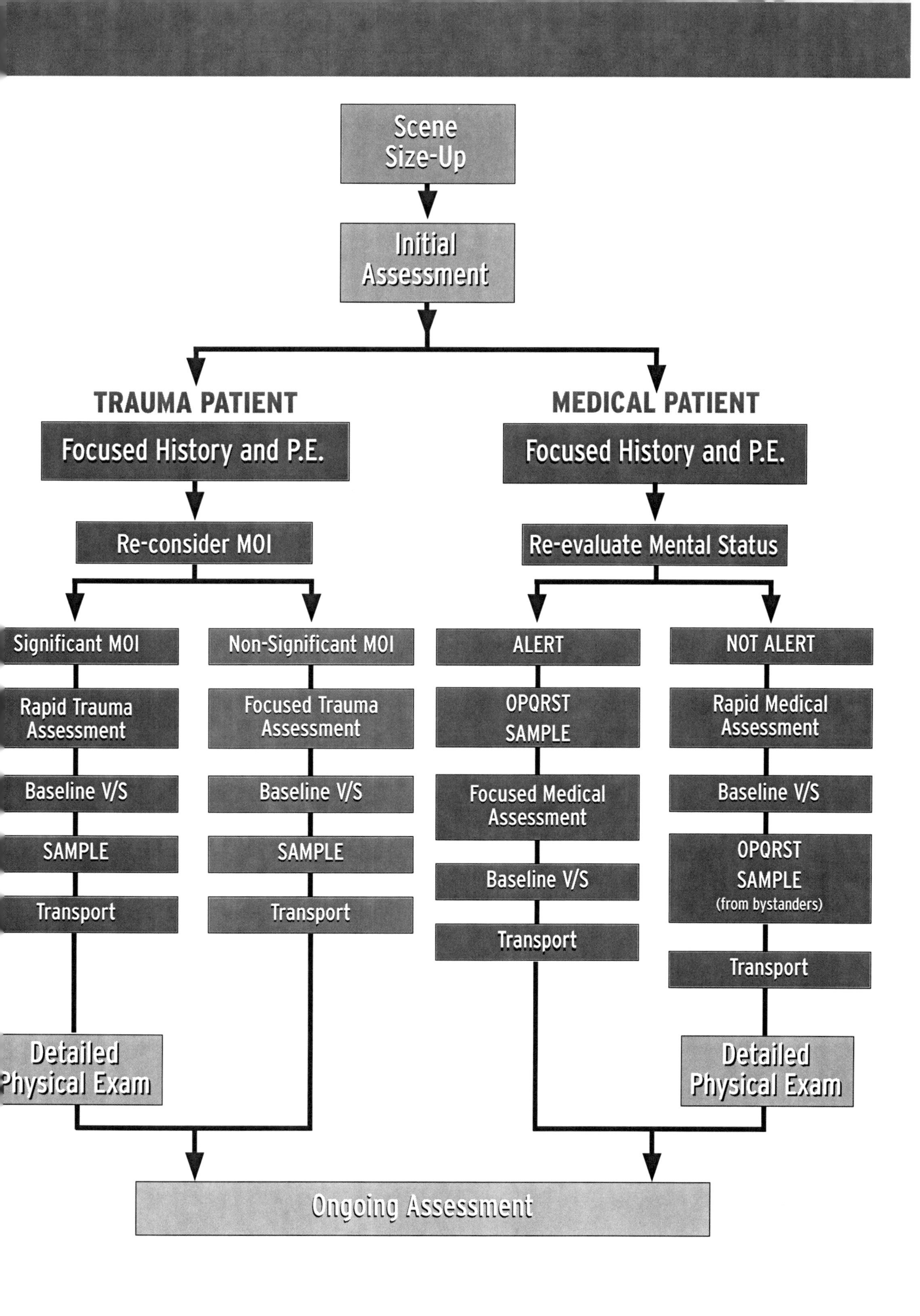
Scene Size-Up
Initial Assessment
TRAUMA PATIENT
Focused History and P.E.
Re-consider MOI
Significant MOI
Rapid Trauma Assessment
Baseline V/S
SAMPLE
Transport
Detailed Physical Exam
Non-Significant MOI
Focused Trauma Assessment
Baseline V/S
SAMPLE
Transport
MEDICAL PATIENT
Focused History and P.E.
Re-evaluate Mental Status
ALERT
OPQRST
SAMPLE
Focused Medical Assessment
Baseline V/S
Transport
NOT ALERT
Rapid Medical Assessment
Baseline V/S
OPQRST
SAMPLE
(from bystanders)
Transport
Detailed Physical Exam
Ongoing Assessment

Printed in the United States
210113BV00001B/139-330/P

9 780763 776640